REAL
Results

with
Karl Henry

THE ULTIMATE HEALTH AND FITNESS GUIDE

BLACKWATER PRESS

Blackwater Press Ltd.
1–5 North Frederick Street, Dublin 1
jloconnor@eircom.net

© Karl Henry, 2010

Edited by: Claire Rourke, Bookends Publishing

Design, layout and cover: Liz White Designs

Studio photography by: Lili Forberg

ISBN 978-0-9563541-9-8

Printed in the Republic of Ireland.

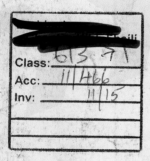

A CIP catalogue record for this book is available from the British Library.

The author and publisher gratefully acknowledge the following for permission to reproduce photographs:

Dreamstime: Liette Parent, Marc Dietrich, Stuart Corlett, Rafal Glebowski, Csaba Fikker, Elena Weber. **Getty Images:** WireImage, Getty Images, FilmMagic. **Inpho Sports Photography:** Inpho/Getty Images, Inpho/Cathal Noonan, Inpho/Dan Sheridan. **SXC images:** Gary Scot, Benjamin Earwicker, Jean Scheijen, Vivek Chugh, Dave Kennard. **iStockPhoto**.

Every effort has been made to contact all copyright holders, if any material used in this book has been reproduced without permission, we would like to rectify this in future editions and encourage owners of copyright material not acknowledged to contact us.

CONTENTS

Introduction

Nutrition

Exercise

Motivation

Acknowledgements

This is a list I have dreamed of writing many times, at both high and low points in my life, an eternal dream that I am delighted to say has come true.

To my mum, dad and brother Cathal: Thanks for your patience and unquestioning faith and support in whatever crazy challenge I come up with. I couldn't do it without knowing that I have you all behind me. Thanks for instilling in me the belief that failure is not a bad thing that reaching for the stars is worth the risk, for being there when I have fallen, and helping me to recharge and reach for my next goal. This book is the product of that faith, trust, love, patience and belief.

To Noel and Niamh at NK Management: You saw something in me all those years ago that made you take a chance. Without your help, not a single word would have made it to print, you both have helped me to fulfil my dreams and to look at new ones, believing that I have what it takes to make them come true. We are an incredible team.

To John, Paula, Claire and Liz: What can I say to you all? You have taken the words and created more than I ever could have imagined at the beginning of this journey. This book will help to spread the message of health – real health – helping people not just to lose weight but to help save lives. Thanks to you all for seeing my dream and producing something of which we can all be so proud.

To my clients: You all are the foundations, the building blocks, that every success has come from. Without your commitment, trust, hard work and belief in yourselves, I would not be writing this book.

To Christy: You've been there from the start, encouraging, helping, listening and singing. You continue to inspire, go raibh maith agait.

To my friends: No matter what, you are there to listen, support, laugh and help. No matter how long I disappear for when I'm training or working, I can always pick up the phone knowing that there will be an answer. Cheers guys.

To Jean: Well doctor, what a team we are – a mutual trust and support that knows no limits, no distance and no boundaries. Tá mé chomh doirte sin duit.

To all those that I can't mention directly, go raibh míle maith again.

Karl Henry

September 2010

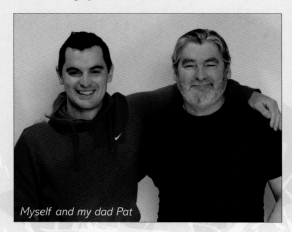

Myself and my dad Pat

Introduction

Look around you. This beautiful nation of ours is heavier and unhealthier than ever before. Yet there is so much confusion about how and what is healthy – from fad diets to vibrating machines, liquid food plans to 30-minute workouts.

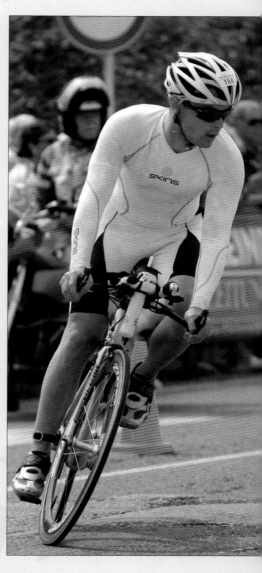

In the next 200 pages, you will find, for the first time, the real way to get healthy, whether it's weight loss, fitness or all-round health that you are aiming for, anyone of any age will find everything they are looking for in this book. My passion in life is to show everyone the way to health – no quick fixes, no crazy diets, nothing that will damage your body in the long run, just pure and simple health.

The secrets and experiences I have learned in my career to help get my clients in the best shape of their lives for movies, tours, photo shoots, weddings, parties, dresses and every other situation that you can imagine, I will share with you in this book. All the mistakes I have made when training for events are here too – so that you don't have to make them.

Many trainers find it hard to associate and identify with those they are trying to help, because they have an elite background in sport – I, however, don't. I lost weight myself, got fit, then progressed into completing marathons and ironman triathlons. I have to continue to eat well and exercise and learn, pushing my body to do these events so that I can prove to my clients and the public that they can do it too, that *you* can do anything you put your mind to.

The following quotation by Theodore Roosevelt is one that has helped me. It sums up my own approach to life and I hope it will help kick start yours …

'It is not the critic who counts; not the man who points out how the strong man stumbles, or where the doer of deeds could have done them better. The credit belongs to the man who is actually in the arena, whose face is marred by dust and sweat and blood, who strives valiantly; who errs and comes short again and again; because there is not effort without error and shortcomings; but who does actually strive to do the deed; who knows the great enthusiasm, the great devotion, who spends himself in a worthy cause, who at the best knows in the end the triumph of high achievement and who at the worst, if he fails, at least he fails while daring greatly. So that his place shall never be with those cold and timid souls who know neither victory nor defeat.'

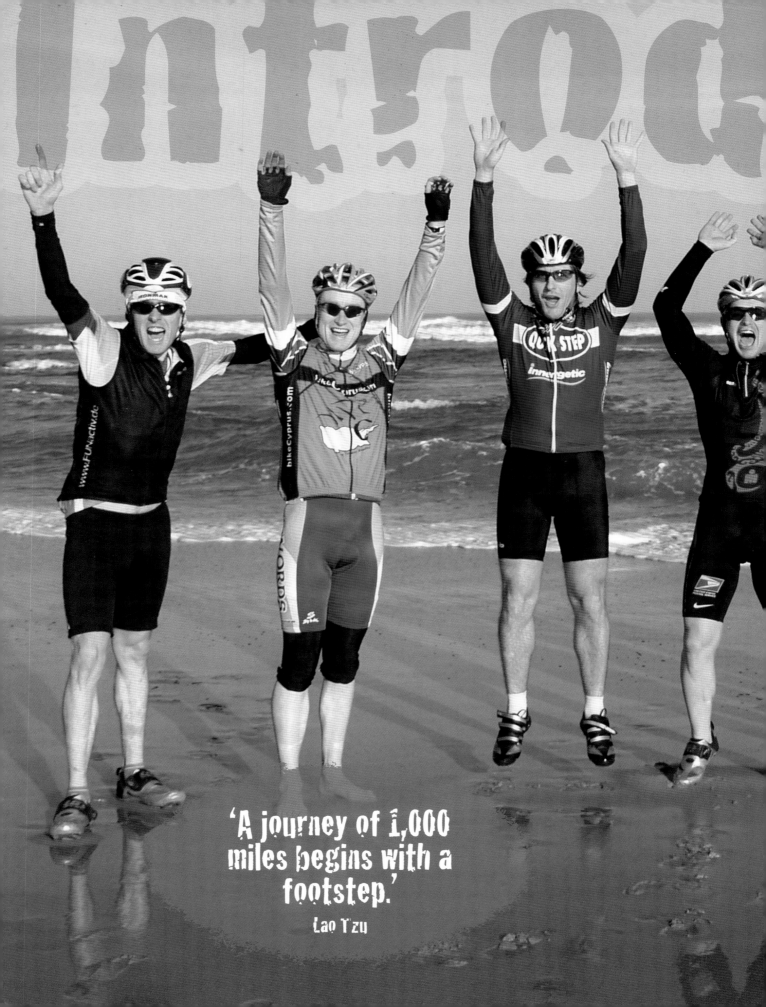

'A journey of 1,000 miles begins with a footstep.'

Lao Tzu

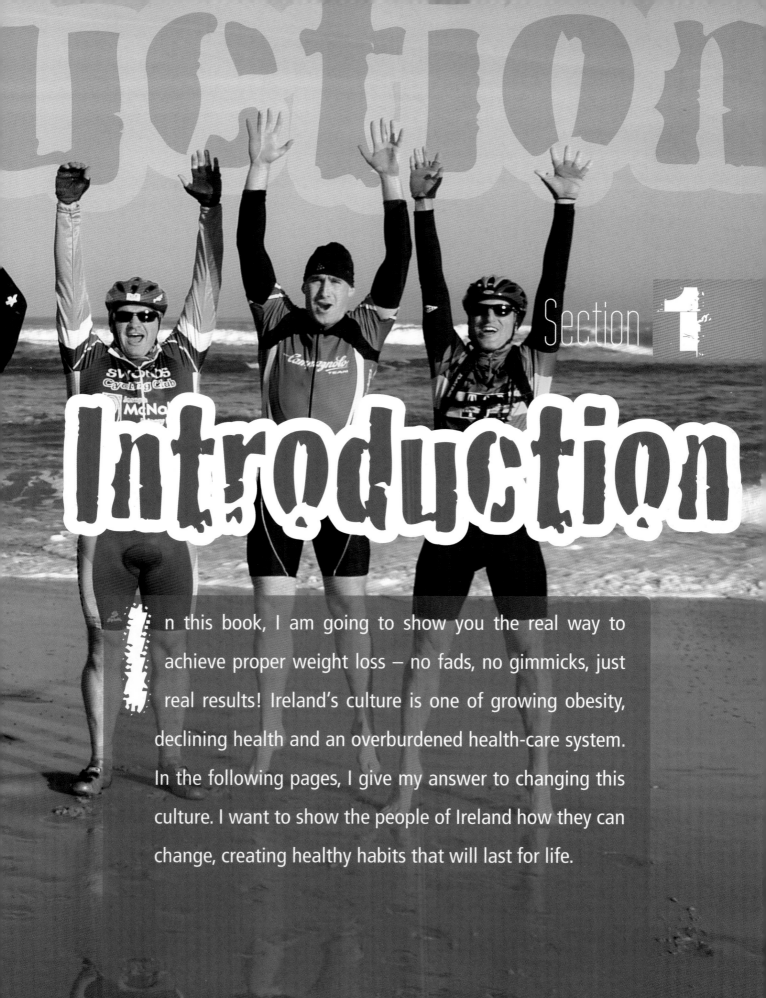

Introduction

n this book, I am going to show you the real way to achieve proper weight loss – no fads, no gimmicks, just real results! Ireland's culture is one of growing obesity, declining health and an overburdened health-care system. In the following pages, I give my answer to changing this culture. I want to show the people of Ireland how they can change, creating healthy habits that will last for life.

Welcome to the first step to a new you!

 Did You Know?

Irish Obesity Statistics

▷ 2 in 5 children are now overweight or obese.

▷ Weight-related issues cost the government €4 billion per year.

▷ Over the past 6 years, Ireland has increased its obesity rate by 30%, with 1 in 8 obese.

▷ 1 in 3 people are overweight.

▷ 2,500 deaths each year are directly caused by obesity, with obesity being the indirect cause in many more.

My company motto has always been: 'No gimmicks, no fads, just real results.' I will make the whole area of weight loss and exercise easy to understand, cutting out the confusing jargon that makes it so difficult for you to reach your goals. I will analyse all those quick fixes that you have tried before in order to lose weight, showing you why they didn't work and also showing you all the tips and tricks that I have learned over the past ten years as I developed my business into Ireland's premier health company.

One of the reasons for our success is that we provide sensible, effective and real solutions to the factors that are gripping Ireland and making the Irish grow heavier and heavier each year.

Whether you are starting from the beginning or super fit and looking to make small changes to improve your racing, you will find everything you need in this book. I have made the journey from being the person who was always last around the laps in training, the person who carried weight through school and into college. I wear T-shirts and clothes now that I could never have worn when I was younger. When I first started running, I could run about 5 kilometres, I now run ultra-marathons that are 63 kilometres.

How other countries are tackling obesity

▷ Australia has banned advertising for food aimed at children under 14.

▷ The Netherlands has banned advertising for food aimed at children under 12.

▷ Sweden has banned the use of cartoons for food marketing.

My name is Liz, I am a forty-two-year-old wife and mother of a six year old, who was born with a chronic illness. In spite of this, I am in the best shape of my life.

When my daughter was born, I put all my energy into her as she required a great deal of care. Though I smoked a lot, I tried to eat healthily and do a little bit of exercise. It was not always possible to keep on top of everything, as a mother the only person whose needs were not being met were mine. There was rarely time for me.

As my daughter became older and I hit my forties, things changed. She became a little bit hardier and I started to feel the onset of the middle-age spread. The changes to my body were huge – the round belly, bingo wings and love handles – but I refused to give into it. I physically might be forty-two but I feel much younger.

I remember standing in a dressing room and it had mirrors on every wall. I could see my body through 360 degrees and was shocked by what I saw – it had been a long time since I had seen my body properly. I left depressed, upset and did not buy a single thing. I did not like my body but knew that only I could change things. It was *the* turning point.

First, I gave up the cigarettes and stopped using them as a crutch because I was stressed, then I found a personal trainer, one hour a week, one to one. I had been in weight watchers since I was twenty, went to the gym, did all the faddy diets but nothing had worked. I now realise there is no quick fix or easy solution. Yet, it is not rocket science, tighten your food, do more exercise and drink more water. Simple changes that mean a lot and I feel so much better. I am hydrated for the first time in my life.

I look forward to my one hour per week with my trainer, who pushes me to my limits. I work hard and we have built up a good relationship – we talk about absolutely everything. He tells me to get walks in between the sessions, keep my diet tight and I feel great.

My routine is built around my daily life, work, school runs, etc. A nurse once told me if I do not look after myself, I am no use to anyone else. No truer words have been spoken, I now have the stamina to look after my family's needs.

I feel energetic, confident, less stressed, fit and happy.

I have become the real me, the person I want to be at last.

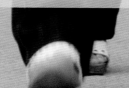

Throughout this book, I am going to share with you all that I have learned, forget all those big Latin words that nobody understands, all they do is massage the experts' egos, as they turn you off the whole idea of exercise.

In this book, my aim is to show you just how easy it is to exercise, to break down all those barriers that have stopped you so far. I won't be lecturing you or nagging you, I will simply be presenting the facts and letting you make your own mind. You will find tips and tricks that I have learned from my experience in the industry, I have made all the mistakes so that you don't have to.

First things first. Listed below are some words that you will be seeing quite often and that it is important you understand.

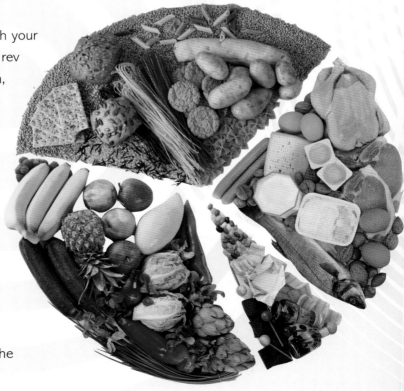

▸ **Metabolism:** This is the rate at which your body burns calories. It's the very same as a rev counter in a car, the higher your metabolism, the more calories you burn. We all have a different metabolic rate and can speed it up through exercise and eating healthily.

▸ **Calorie:** This is simply a unit of energy. It enables us to know how much energy certain food types are giving us. The different nutrients all contain a different number of calories.

▸ **Dieting:** This normally consists of a restriction of certain foods for short-term weight loss, resulting in weight gain when the restricted foods are reintroduced.

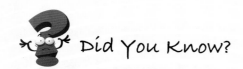

Did You Know?

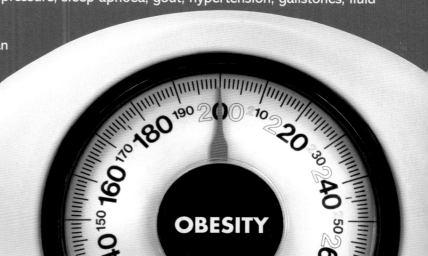

Why am I so concerned with tackling the obesity epidemic gripping Ireland? Well let's look at what being overweight does to us.

▷ It increases the risk of heart attacks, strokes and cancer.

▷ It increases the risk of arthritis, osteoporosis, type-2 diabetes, depression and acne.

▷ It leads to high cholesterol, high blood pressure, sleep apnoea, gout, hypertension, gallstones, fluid retention, IBS, anxiety and migraines.

▷ It leads to a poorer quality of life and an earlier death.

▷ Being overweight reduces concentration, reduces work productivity, increases fatigue and leads to poor self-confidence.

▷ It gives us higher stress levels and poorer relationships.

Are there enough reasons there?

What if I told you that Ireland has the highest rate of childhood obesity in Europe and the second highest in the world? Obesity in Ireland costs the government an estimated €4 billion every year (www.dohc.ie). The Americanisation of Irish society has led to an obesity epidemic that will eclipse America's. We are no longer shocked by what we see when we go on holidays. You can blame the government, the schools or anyone that you want but, guess what, the responsibility lies with you.

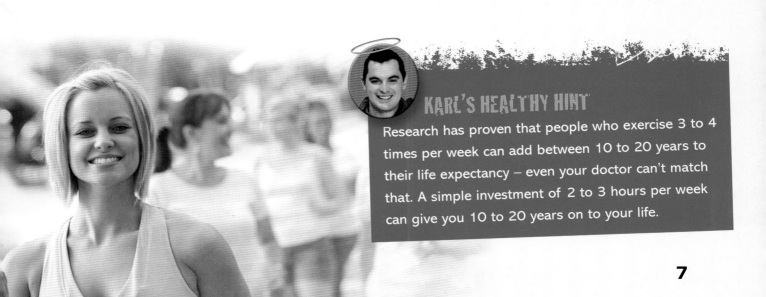

KARL'S HEALTHY HINT

Research has proven that people who exercise 3 to 4 times per week can add between 10 to 20 years to their life expectancy – even your doctor can't match that. A simple investment of 2 to 3 hours per week can give you 10 to 20 years on to your life.

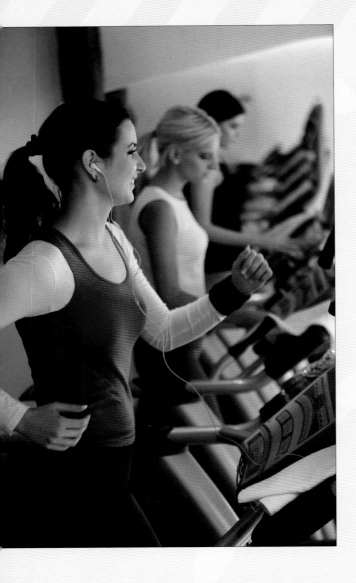

Get moving

One of the greatest threats to health is not age, it is inactivity. By sitting more and moving less, we are getting older faster! Every year, people spend thousands of euros, trying that year's latest quick fix to help them look and feel younger – but by getting out and exercising more, you can begin to reverse the ageing process. Let's have a look how:

▸ Regular exercise increases blood flow to the brain, stimulating the brain and slowing down the degeneration of the central nervous system.

▸ Exercise increases the strength and tone of your muscles, helping you to look leaner, stronger and fitter as you age.

▸ By exercising, you will have improved lung and heart function, ensuring that your body is under less stress every day just to function.

▸ By exercising, you will have lower body fat, especially important in men as it has great benefits for the heart.

▸ Exercising in the fresh air is one of the best ways to revitalise your skin and clear away the dead skin cells, leaving you refreshed. I often get asked how my skin is so good, the answer is simple, a good diet and regular exercise out in the open air!

▸ By exercising, your bones become stronger, reducing your risk of getting conditions such as osteoporosis, arthritis and bone-density disorders – and it reduces their impact if you already have them.

▸ Many medical conditions, if not all, that require medication can be improved by exercise. I have numerous clients who have reduced, or stopped, taking all of their medication as a direct result of doing the exercises in this book. More and more doctors are waking up to the concept of exercise prescription to solve common problems rather than tablet taking.

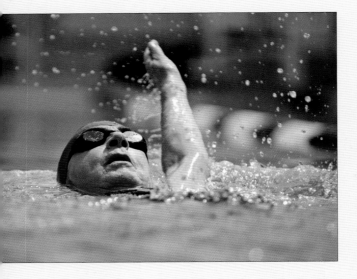

Age and exercise

TEST YOUR SKIN AGE

Simply pinch the skin on the back of your hand between the thumb and the forefinger for 5 seconds and time how long it takes to flatten out completely.

Average rates per age:

>50	5 seconds
60 years old	10 to 15 seconds
70 years of age	35 to 55 seconds

Your skin elasticity is a result of the underlying deterioration of the connective tissues, such as collagen and elastin, under your skin's surface.

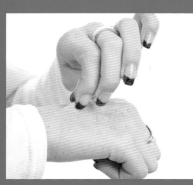

This skin age test will give you an indicator of how old your skin really is, try it now and then try it in 4 weeks time after you have been following my plan – the results will amaze you.

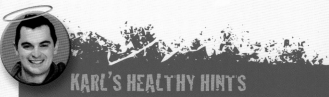
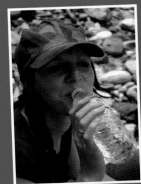

KARL'S HEALTHY HINTS

Karl's five tips for speeding up your metabolism:

▷ Drink more water during the day.

▷ Walk more.

▷ Eat 5 small meals rather than 3 big ones.

▷ Eat a proper nutritious breakfast.

▷ Try to avoid eating large meals after 7 p.m.

Syringe

Diabetes

Pancreas

Obesity

Before we start on the road to fitness, let's look at what happens when your body ages. Do you actually know what is happening to your body as you age? Does your metabolism change or stay the same? Exercise can play a vital role in life at any age, but what exactly does it do? Let's take a look through the different age groups so see what happens to your body.

The decades of health

Teens

In your youth, you learn the habits that you will have for life. It is so essential to open up your mind to exercise and the many benefits that it provides, as well as learning about healthy food and the basics of food preparation. In your teens, you have amazing energy and zest for life as well as a lack of fear that seems to surround people as they grow older. The more skills and sports that you have in your teens, the less likely it is that you will have a weight problem as you get older.

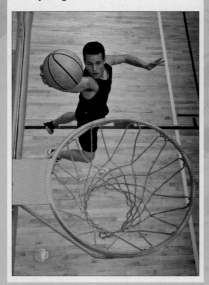

Twenties

When you are in your twenties, your metabolism is at its peak, so, in theory, you should be in the best shape of your life – if your diet and exercise are good! If they are not, however, you may find that you are developing cellulite or man boobs. In your twenties, you can no longer hide the effects of a bad diet I'm afraid.

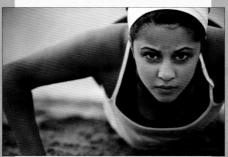

Thirties

In your thirties, your metabolism begins to slow down, causing reduced muscle mass and increased fat content on your body. For most people, their working and family lives have taken over, placing more stress on their time and, before they know it, they have the middle-age spread. That lip of fat around your midsection that was never there before. Suddenly, you will begin to be more affected by moods as stress begins to affect you. The seasonal affective disorder might even appear, where your mood will change with the seasons. For women, the effects of PMS generally become more severe.

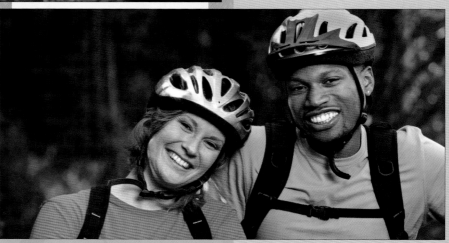

> No matter what age you are, exercise and diet will improve all the issues that arise in the different stages of life!

Forties

Having peaked in your mid-thirties, your bone density is now beginning to decrease steadily. This affects the strength of your bones and their ability to recover from breaks and fractures. Your aerobic system begins to decline, the more sedentary your lifestyle, the faster it will decline. You will have roughly 30 per cent less muscle strength than you did in your twenties and your flexibility will decrease too, making your body less supple.

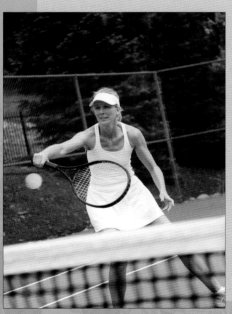

Fifties

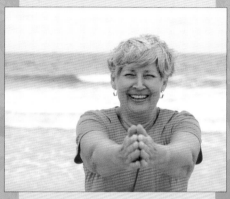

Women in their fifties will have on average 20 per cent less aerobic capacity than they did in their twenties. This can increase the strain on your heart as it has to work harder. Bone density is on the decrease, especially amongst women, as reduced oestrogen levels cause calcium to leak out of the bones. You can lose up to 5 per cent of your bone density every year for up to seven years after menopause. Suddenly, conditions such as osteoporosis and arthritis, from which over 400,000 people in Ireland suffer, could start to develop in your hands, feet, knees or hips.

Sixties +

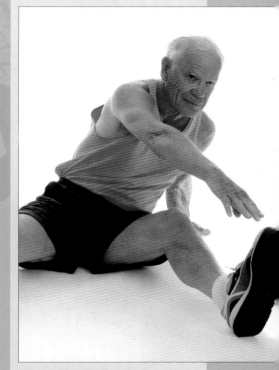

Your metabolism slows down yet again, I am afraid. This means that you burn fewer calories naturally during the day. Your skin ages as the skin cells hold less water, you will have reduced muscle tone and muscle strength. You will also find that you will tire easily and be more affected by the weather, which, in many respects, is due to your metabolism slowing down.

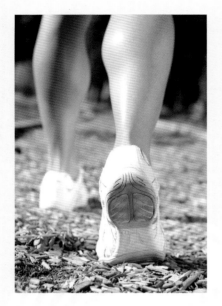

Now that you have read the bad news, let me fill you in on the good news. Every change in your body that happens with age can be improved with even the most simple exercise. Movement in any shape or form will have a huge impact on your health. Conditions such as arthritis and osteoporosis will improve with weight-bearing exercise and your metabolism will actually increase when you exercise. Aerobic exercise, such as walking, will help to reduce stress levels, improve the fitness of your heart, tone your body and so many other things. If you want to stop your bone density from weakening, guess what you should do … exercise!

Using just two water bottles, you can do simple exercises at home that will stop the damaging effects of age that you have read about above, so what are you waiting for! By following the exercises in Chapter 3, you can actually reverse the ageing process – yes I said reverse!

Excuses – I can't exercise because…

Karl's Tips for Success

'I don't measure a man's success by how high he climbs but how high he bounces when he hits bottom.'
General George S. Patton

In my years of working with people, I have heard every excuse in the book about why people can't exercise! However, if you make up your mind to do something and promise yourself and those around you that you will persist until you have reached your goal, despite any road block that may get in your way, you will get there! Simply make a deal with yourself to persist until you reach your goal and, believe me, you will get there. Many of the excuses people have relate to their age. Now that you know age is no excuse, let's look at some of the others.

KARL'S HEALTHY HINT

Treats: Always have one treat day each week where you can eat whatever you want! The latest research from America has proven that, by doing this, you are actually helping to speed up your metabolism as your body has to speed up to burn off all the calories that it isn't used to. It also means that you will stay healthy longer as you aren't cutting out junk food for the rest of your life, something that no one could do! It's all about balance!

There's not enough time

The excuse that I hear most often from people is the fact that they are just too busy to exercise! In reality, exercise doesn't have to always done in the gym. Lifestyles just get busier and busier, that won't change, what you need to do is to add exercise into your life, make it a part of your daily routine. Now I'm not talking about walking a marathon to work, like US fitness guru Bernarr Macfadden used to in the late 1800s, I am simply saying you will be surprised just how big a difference you can make in your life by changing small things. Little changes add up, try some of these changes for a few weeks and see just what a difference they make to your life.

1. No more lifts/escalators: Why not use the stairs from now on? The first time you do, you may be out of breath but, with persistence, you will become fitter and fitter. Each step works the legs, bum and gives you a great workout!

2. Make the office smoke break your exercise break: If you sit a desk a lot during the day, then every hour you should get up and walk around the office for at least five minutes. While your colleagues are having their smoke break, up you get and walk around, adding more movement into your day.

3. Get off that extra stop early: On the way to work or even on the way home, why not get off the stop before your normal one and walk that little bit extra, especially if it's a nice day out. You will find that not only will the walk make you feel better, it will relieve your stress from the day and leave you feeling invigorated.

4. Take the meeting outside: The sun is shining, so why not take that board meeting outside and enjoy it? You may just find that your meeting is more productive too!

5. Leave the SUV at home: If your child's school is close by, well why not walk them to school or even better why not cycle with them to school? Ireland is becoming more and more bike friendly and your kids will love it!

6. Walk to the shops: Just as above, do you really need to drive to the shop just down the road? Remember your trying to get more movement into your day and here is a great way to do it. While it might take you a little longer, are you really in that much of a hurry that you can't take a few extra minutes to walk to the shops?

7. *Just do it*, as the ad says: Sometimes the biggest obstacle in getting more movement into your day is actually doing it. A million excuses will come up and try to stop you, but I promise you, just getting into the routine of doing something is the hardest part. We hate change, but when we are used to it, we suddenly like it. So go on, give it a go!

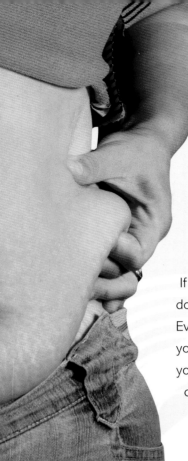

I'm too overweight to start

Many people believe that they are simply too heavy to start exercising and that they simply can't do anything but sit and get heavier, letting life become more and more difficult because of their weight!

Come on guys and girls do you really think this or are you using this as an excuse? No matter what weight you are – 30 stone or 13 – you can achieve equally great results. As we discussed earlier, you just need to progress slowly and safely, so that you build up your fitness gradually.

If you are very overweight and get out of breath easily, then why not try to do a 20-minute walk every day, combined with one set of my exercises? Even with a simple programme like this, you can achieve results, and you will feel better and more positive. This will continue to progress as you get fitter and stronger, showing you the gateway to getting your old self back or creating your new self, getting fit and firm for the first time. The national guidelines on physical activity for Ireland recommend that you get at least 30 minutes of moderate activity a day. For many people that may seem like too much, so why not start off slowly and build it up gradually?

I smoke

In Ireland, 31 per cent of people smoke – that's nearly 1 in 3 people! Nicotine is known to be more addictive than heroin, cocaine, alcohol, cannabis and caffeine, so don't worry if you have failed to give up before, the reason is that it is so addictive.

I'm not going to lecture you on just how bad smoking is, I will simply present you with the facts and let you make up your own mind. Smoking has known links to cancer, heart attacks, blood clots, strokes, ulcers, lung infections and bronchitis. For all you men out there, suffering from impotence, guess what, the level of impotence is 50 per cent higher in men who smoke!

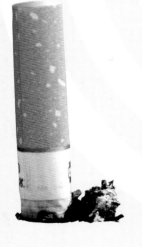

Whatever about your decision to damage your own body, it is even worse for those around you. The next time you are smoking in the car with the windows closed, have a think about what you are doing to your passengers. The smoke inhaled by passive smokers contains 70 per cent more tar and over 100 times more carcinogens (cancer-causing agents) than smoking the cigarette itself – you are causing more damage to those around you than you are to yourself. Some children can be exposed to the equivalent of 150 cigarettes per year through passive smoking!

Real Results

What about those of you who smoke through pregnancy, any ideas of the effects you are having on your baby?

▸ Babies born to smokers tend to be 200g lighter.

▸ By smoking while pregnant, you increase the chance of your baby being premature, stillborn or suffering early death syndrome.

▸ The children of smokers tend to be smaller and less well developed intellectually and emotionally.

▸ Your newborn baby is at an increased risk of respiratory illnesses, such as bronchitis and pneumonia.

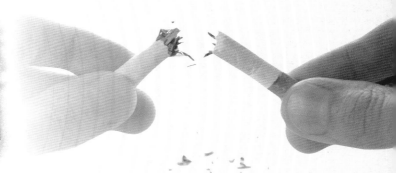

Karl's Tip for Smokers

Try and eat at least 2 oranges a day or 200 mg of a vitamin C supplement, as smoking, even passively, can deplete your vitamin C stores!

These are just some of the facts about smoking, the next time you light up read them again and see what you think.

There are also the financial implications, let's have a look.

An average smoker smokes 22 cigarettes per day.

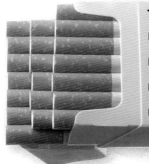

This equals:
▸ €7.15 per day
▸ €50.05 per week
▸ €200.20 per month
▸ €2,400.40 per year

I know it's addictive, but if you truly want to quit, **you can do it!**

Many people fear that they will put on weight if they give up the demon drug as cigarettes act as an appetite suppressant. When you give up smoking, your metabolism slows down and your appetite increases. Listed below are a few tips that will help you to keep that weight off.

▸ Speed up your metabolism through a healthy diet and exercise.

▸ Try to exercise in the morning as it will keep your metabolism higher during the day.

▸ Be positive and reward yourself for every week you manage to stay off the cigarettes.

▸ Drink at least 2 litres of water per day to keep your body hydrated.

▸ Apples are full of antioxidants that will help to undo the damage done to your lungs, so eat plenty.

▸ Don't crash diet, your metabolism can then increase naturally.

Mythbusting

The whole area of fitness and health is clouded in false facts that do nothing but confuse, so let's take a look at some of the myths that are out there and see if there is any truth in them.

Muscle is heavier than fat

This is one thing that comes up all the time when I do my lectures around the country and I am afraid that it is indeed a myth – 1 pound of muscle weighs exactly the same as 1 pound of fat. They both weigh a pound.

What is different is the *density* of the two. The next time you are in your butcher's, ask him for 1 pound of muscle and 1 pound of fat – you'll be amazed at what comes out, the pound of fat looks so much bigger as there is more mass; the pound of muscle is smaller and denser, yet they both weigh a pound!

It is also true that muscle cannot turn into fat or visa versa. Muscle that isn't used becomes soft, it simply loses its tone. Fat may begin to store close to that area because of a poor diet and lack of activity, but they are two very different entities. When you start exercising, the fat will begin to disappear and the muscle will become more toned.

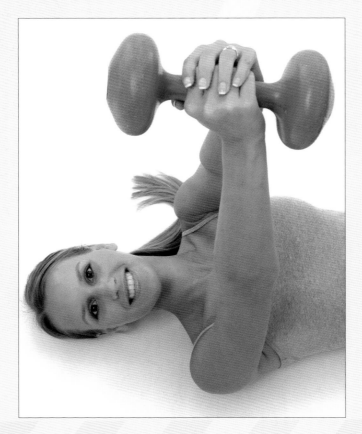

Weights will make you bulky

This is another preconception on the market, especially amongst women who feel that by touching a weight, they will develop huge muscles. Weights done correctly will not make you bigger or develop big muscles. Higher rep workouts, such as the ones in this book, will tone and sculpt your muscles like no other workout, giving you a firm, toned body. Keeping the weights light will ensure that you keep that feminine shape that you want to work towards. When thinking of weight workouts, women often think of the scary, grunting men in the local gyms who hog the mirrors and lift big weights, this, I am glad to say, is not something you have to do! Leave those men to massage their egos by doing the wrong technique and follow my plans to get you into great shape.

Real Results

Cardiovascular workouts alone are the best way to lose fat

While running, walking and cycling will help to burn fat and calories, the best way to lose fat is through a combination of three things: a good diet, resistance workouts and cardiovascular workouts. This combination will give you the best results of your life, rather than concentrating on just one element on its own. All too often, your local gym programme will consist of just cardiovascular work on a machine, this has nothing to do with the benefits of the machine,

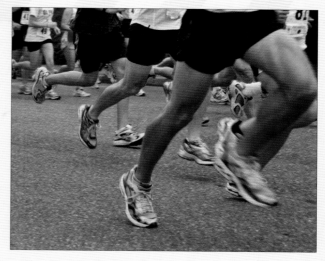

it simply means that the gym staff don't have to work with you as much, and can leave you on your own. To get the best results, you need to add in the resistance workouts, so no more pure cardio sessions in the gym!

You can spot reduce one area

Your body is an amazing machine that can adapt to any environment. It cannot, however, specifically reduce weight from one area. No matter what marketing jargon you read, I am here to tell you it simply cannot be done. Your body will dictate where the weight loss occurs, all you can do is ensure you do full body workouts that work every body part so that you lose weight and inches all over.

Sit-ups will give you a flat stomach

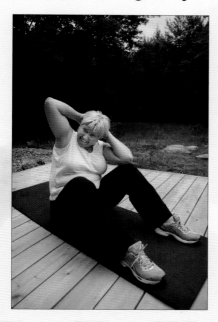

This is one of my favourites, again it is a total myth. We all have a six-pack, you, me and every other person out there. What makes us all different is the layer of fat that covers it. Guess what? All those hundreds of sit-ups will strengthen your abdominal muscles if you are weak there, but will do absolutely nothing to shift that fat around your waist – nothing at all. Eating the right food and cardiovascular sessions are the key ways to shift that muffin top, not sit-ups! In fact, if you overdo your sit-ups, you can make your waist wider and thicker as the muscle just begins to expand.

Eating less will help you lose weight

An all too common reason that people don't exercise, or tend to fall off the wagon and go back to eating junk food when they have started, is that they stop losing weight. No matter what they do, it simply will not shift! This is one of the most frustrating parts of weight loss and the one that generally signals the end of someone's healthy eating. Well let's look at why this happens.

Your body adapts itself to the environment that it finds itself in. If you sit all day, your body will adapt to that, if you are active, it will adapt to that too. But here is the catch, your body has a rate of adaptation. What this means is that you will rapidly adapt to a new environment in the first few weeks, but, after a couple of weeks, you will see less and less change.

Ever wonder why people recommend that you change your gym plan every six weeks? This is the reason. Your body will adapt to a new programme very quickly but after four weeks, there really is very little adaptation. Most people don't change their plan and stop going to the gym as they aren't seeing any results. When I train with my clients, every session is different – no two sessions the same. This means that their bodies are constantly adapting and it is one of the reasons why my results are so good with my clients.

By changing your programmes on a session or weekly basis, you will see much faster results, and you will stop the weight plateau that causes so much grief. Aim to change your routes every week for your walks, etc. because if you continue to do the same route, you won't be seeing any changes!

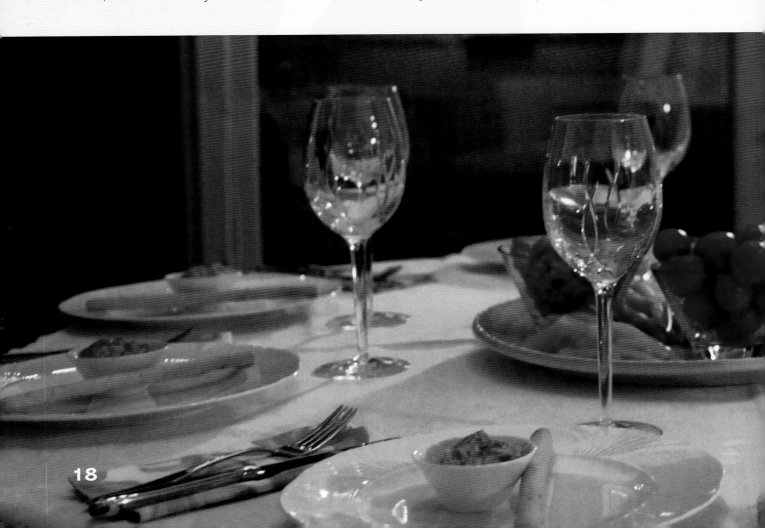

Sometimes bodies hold on to weight for a few weeks for no reason, then continue to lose it again after that, I have seen this time and time again and here persistence is key. Just keep working hard, keep eating the right food and you will lose weight.

In one instance, a client that I was working with had failed to lose weight for two weeks, despite being put on a low-calorie diet of 1,200 calories by a nutritionist. The nutritionist who was working with her insisted that she reduce her calorie intake even further to 600 calories per day. I knew that this wouldn't work and recommended that she actually increase her calorie intake. We agreed to try both methods. After the week of the low calorie diet, the client had, again, lost no weight. After the week returning to a normal calorie consumption of around 1,800 calories, the client shifted 3 pounds, a result that was baffling to everyone but me.

Your body has a self-protection mechanism, if it feels that it is being underfed, then it will hold on to weight to protect itself. It generally will hold on to fat as fat has more calories and is a better source of insulation than protein. If your calorie intake is too low in your diet, then this is what may happen. By increasing the calories to a normal intake, the body's metabolism returned and, hey presto, the client lost weight. It may sound very strange but in order to lose weight healthily, you need to eat plenty of food, just the right food!

The lesson to learn from this is the fact that if your weight does stabilise, try to change your workout, persist with your food and if you are eating too little, then increase your intake of healthy food.

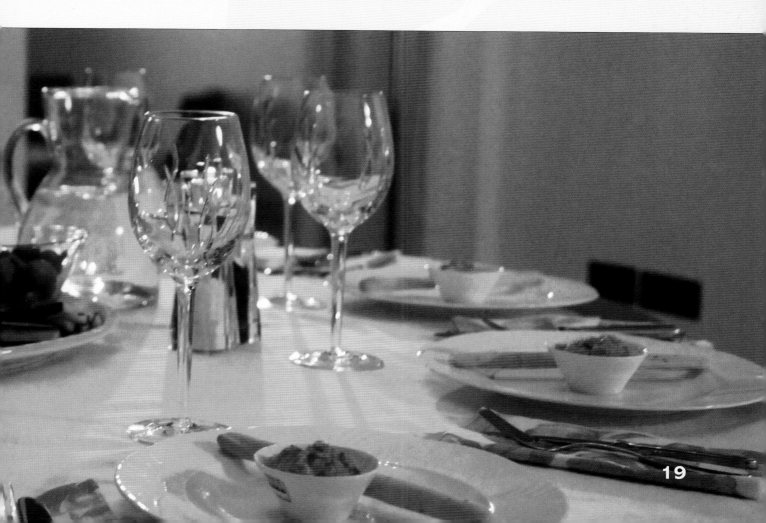

Common medical conditions and how exercise can help

MODERN LIFE AND WEIGHT GAIN	
Transportation	**At Home**
▸ Rise in car ownership. ▸ Increase in driving shorter distances. ▸ Decrease in walking or cycling.	▸ Increase in the use of modern appliances (e.g. microwaves, dishwashers, washing machines, vacuum cleaners). ▸ Increase in ready-made foods and ingredients for cooking. ▸ Increase in television viewing, and computer and video game use. ▸ Decrease in manual labour. ▸ Increase in consumption of convenience foods that contribute to obesity. ▸ Decrease in time spent on more active recreational pursuits.

Exercise has an enormous role to play in both the prevention and management of nearly all medical conditions. One of the easiest and most common indicators for cardiovascular problems is the size of your waist – the smaller the size, the lower your risk factor.

Exercise and diet have a direct role to play in this. Equally important is the fact that exercise can help you to manage a medical condition better, improve your quality of life and often reduce the amount of medication that you are taking.

I have had many clients over the years who have had their medication reduced because they have started to exercise. The medical profession is now coming around to the fact that exercise prescription is the key to treating and helping many medical conditions, in conjunction with medication. I truly believe that it is the way forward for the health

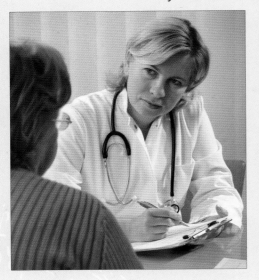

system as a whole, a combination of better food, more exercise and quality medication will get patients better, back on track and back into their lives.

I work with many doctors – I only wish that it was more – and all agree that one of the main benefits of a multifaceted programme like this is the great domino affect it has. A patient's improved diet and exercise regime not only improves his life, but the lives of those around him. The more people we can educate to this way of thinking, the healthier this nation will be.

As we get older, we build up barriers around ourselves, telling ourselves that we can't do things. This is also true if we have a

Real Results

medical condition. The norm is to accept that you have the condition and that you can't exercise. But the reality is that no matter what medical condition you have, there is a form of exercise that will suit you – it is your mind that is stopping you from doing it. It is just as important for you to be healthy, as someone without the condition.

All too often, I see people give up their training when they are newly diagnosed with a medical condition. Through demotivation and, sometimes, through fear, people fall off the wagon and find it hard to get back on. Doctors and medical consultants should be working with gyms and fitness professionals to help get their patients back on track, providing the support, help and sometimes a slightly firm hand to get their patients moving, exercising and working towards a goal.

I have seen amazing results not just in the motivation of my clients, but the health benefits, psychological benefits, confidence benefits and, in many cases, the actual reduction of medication.

I hate being told that someone can't do something or that something can't be done, where there is a will there is a way, a refusal to not take no for an answer is often the key in getting yourself back on track. Push yourself, your partner, your gym, your doctor and anyone else in your life to give you the support that you are going to need to get back exercising because often we lose sight that we are, in fact, consumers.

We have a right to service and shouldn't be afraid to demand it whether we are in our GP's surgery or in the local gym.

Back pain

Back pain is one of the most uncomfortable problems to get as it affects everything you do. Our lives have changed with the booming economy and we sit down more than we used to – in our cars, in our jobs and at home while watching our super huge plasma televisions.

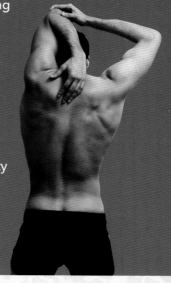

I have clients who travel from all around the country to see me in relation to improving their back trouble. Below are my secrets to helping them (and you) solve the pain.

Get a phone book or a book of similar size and place in under your feet. Now while you are working aim to have one foot on the book at all times. This takes the strain off your lower back because your hamstrings aren't strained. Try it for one week, I guarantee you will find your pain is lessened.

If you are in the car a lot, then I recommend you get a back support. Most car seats have poor back support so you slump in the seat. Try to walk at least fifteen or twenty minutes at the end of the day too, or try to swim, as these two exercises will loosen out your tight muscles after a hard day.

For all you spa lovers out there, massage is obviously great for your lower back too and it's a great way to treat yourself.

I come from a family who all have back pain, my dad has had two discs removed, my mum has a twisted pelvis and both my brother and myself have curvatures in our spines. So, needless to say, we are well used to dealing with back problems.

Back pain initially starts with bad posture – these two things are always linked – and normally begins in schools, where children have to carry bags that are too heavy. This forces children to crouch forward, damaging their lower back in the process. Another way in which bad posture develops is in school gyms amongst teenage boys, who want to be the biggest and strongest and tend to curve their shoulders to make them look more muscular. If this is not addressed, it can lead to serious back problems in later life.

Another source of back pain is not stretching. This isn't too noticeable when we are young but as we grow older, tight hamstrings are one of the most common causes of lower back pain. Over 90 per cent of people I have worked with, who have back pain, have very tight hamstrings. Exercising using yoga or Pilates is a great way to become more flexible fast and the stretches on pages 138–142 are also a great way to loosen up.

Your job can obviously be a prime cause of back pain too. I can now almost tell what people do based on their posture. If you sit at a desk all day or at a computer, then you tend to crouch forward with inadequate padding in the seat to support your body.

Stress

How can you take care of others if you can't take of yourself?

We are now, more than ever, a nation of mortgage slaves, stressed out of our minds from a concoction of traffic, work and the overall pace of life – and we're not showing any signs of getting better. Stress is one of the leading causes of most medical conditions and if you find that you are badly affected by it, then it's time to do something about it before it affects your health even more.

Stress causes:

▷ insomnia

▷ depression

▷ weakened immune system

▷ heart disease

▷ high blood pressure

▷ migraine

▷ difficulty in socialising

Stress causes so many things: insomnia, depression, a weakened immune system, heart disease, high blood pressure, migraines and can lead to a difficulty socialising.

Do these symptoms seem familiar to you? Well, you're not alone.

With out modern lifestyles, it is easy to let stress get a grip on your day. Sitting in traffic, being squashed on trains and buses, dealing with difficult work colleagues, and money and relationship worries – all areas of our lives can be affected by stress. But there are ways to help alleviate some of it.

Become an early riser. Get out of bed half an hour earlier in the morning and beat the traffic! If you get the bus, train or the Dart, why not get off a few stops early and walk the rest of the way to work, you will be amazed at how chilled you are when you get to work. When you're in work, take a five-minute break from your desk, a 'stroll break'. It's very easy, leave everything at your desk, including your mobile, and just walk around for five minutes, preferably outside.

Don't sit at your desk during your lunch break, turn off your phone for 20 minutes and just interact with the people around you, or sit quietly on your own. Again, you will be mentally refreshed, ready to go for the rest of the day.

Keep a to-do list and, at the start of each day, write down the things you need to get done, just tick off the tasks as the day goes on. If you don't finish everything on your list, then chill – just carry it over into the following day.

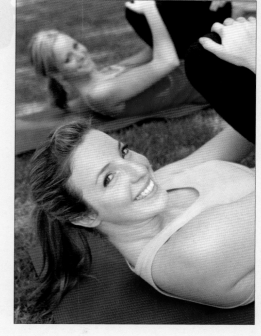

At the end of the day, why not go to the gym or for a walk? Exercise is the best form of stress relief there is, producing endomorphs, which are also called the happy hormones. These make you feel good, and are best produced by exercise. Exercise classes can also be a great way to off load that stress too, see if there are any close to your workplace, so that you can miss the traffic jams and then go home relaxed.

Obviously, your diet plays a hugely important role in how you manage stress. Sometimes, people eat emotionally to deal with a stressful situation, often leading to rapid weight gain over a short period of time. Even during your day, the fluid that you drink will have a profound impact on how you deal with stress. Basically, in my opinion, the more coffee you drink, the less well you will deal with stress. Water and fresh juices are much healthier for your body and enable you to deal with the stress around you better.

Depression

I have witnessed the benefits that exercise and an improved diet can have on people suffering with depression and other mood-related conditions.

Exercise produces endorphins, the happy hormones, which give you a sense of exultation after you exercise. This is one of the most natural tools the body has to improve depression. I know that exercise may be the last thing you want to do, but reach out to others, to gym staff or trainers and be a consumer, look for some assistance because I can guarantee that they will get enormous satisfaction from helping you.

The other important element to consider is the food you eat. Foods high in sugar will naturally lead to mood swings, because when you eat this food, you will be on a serious high for 45 minutes after which, you will be very low as your blood sugar levels reduce – unfortunately this happens with most processed foods in the Irish diet. The food plans on pages 58–64 will free you from this dreaded sugar cycle and give you more constant levels of energy throughout the day.

Arthritis

Every pound that we are over weight results in over 8 pounds of extra pressure on our joints. So it is no wonder that over 10 per cent of the Irish population (400,000 people) suffer from arthritis. Now I am not suggesting that all these cases are caused by obesity, but it is definitely a major factor, along with age, being female, genetics and pre-existing joint injuries. Obesity in linked with osteoarthritis of the hand, hip, back and knee.

If you have arthritis, there are so many things that you can do to reduce the pain – and sitting around in your favourite chair isn't one of them. Gentle exercise, such as walking or swimming, will reduce the joint pain – it will also increase your muscle strength, your flexibility and your overall fitness.

Diabetes

Most people think that if they have diabetes they can't exercise – but this is a myth! People with diabetes can do almost any exercise, just start slowly and build up your fitness levels over time. Moderate exercise causes a glucose uptake at roughly 20 times the normal rate, it is only with intense exercise that you may need insulin after your workouts.

One area to keep an eye on when exercising is your feet, as people with diabetes are more susceptible to infections. Always dry your feet after showers, use moisturiser and athlete's foot spray if required.

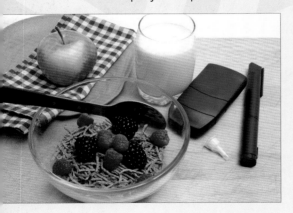

Aim to have carbohydrates before and after your workout to get the best results from your training and to keep your blood sugars constant.

There are some things to look out for though. Always ensure that you warm up and cool down for a safe effective workout. Don't exercise if your blood sugar or ketone level is very high. Try to get into a regular routine to avoid the risk of hypoglycaemia. Be careful about exercising when your medicine is reaching its peak effect. If you feel shaky/weak/confused or have headaches, then stop straight away.

Multiple Sclerosis (MS)

I am lucky enough to be part of a group of experts that travels to each province, talking to people with MS in workshops designed to motivate and inform them that they can exercise and let them know the benefits it can bring.

Like other medical conditions, MS should not stop you from training. No matter what form of MS you have, or what stage it has developed to, if you are willing to put in the time, you can achieve great results. Walking, swimming, yoga and Pilates are all forms of exercise that you can do.

The greatest fear when exercising with MS is that it will trigger a relapse. In a recent Irish survey, where MS patients on exercise plans were tracked over several months, 1 per cent suffered a relapse. The MS Association of Ireland runs fantastic classes around the country that were part of this survey and have had great success with them.

Exercising will improve your bone density, your muscle strength and tone, your mental function, your bowel movements, will lower any levels of depression and mood swings and will improved your management of MS.

However, at even the slightest sign of dizziness, nausea, pins and needles or any other symptom, sit down and take it easy, take some water on board and recover. Regulate your temperature. When you exercise, your body temperature goes up, it is important for MS patients, to monitor this. Moderation is the key.

If you suffer from cold limbs, get some winter training clothing such as that by Under Armour or Canterbury, which are a snug fit that can be worn under your clothes.

Asthma

With gradual adaptation to a training plan, exercising with asthma can be safe and enjoyable. To be safe when exercising, you should always have your inhaler with you, and also try to avoid training alone (or always carry a mobile phone). The next point is especially important, breathe through your nose as this will help moisten the air, making life so much easier for your lungs. This is especially true in winter, when the air is cold, but should be done even during the summer. When you are not exercising, try breathing through your nose as it will make a huge difference to your asthma.

Exercising with asthma

▷ If you are just starting out with your training, keep the resistance light and build it up over the course of a few weeks. Start with basic exercises, like bench presses and squats, and build up your strength.

▷ Ensure you take sufficient breaks in between each exercise to enable your lungs to recover. This is essential as you don't want your breathing rate to go too high, you should always be able to talk.

▷ Asthmatics can undertake any form of exercise – the important factor is your breathing rate, as you get fitter, you will find that you can do more.

▷ Passive forms of exercise, such as yoga, tai chi and Pilates, can also help with this by teaching you how to use more of your lungs to breath.

Most of us only use 40 per cent of our lung capacity and these forms of exercise can teach you how to use much more.

▷ I always ask clients of mine who have asthma to reduce the number of dairy products in their diet, as this will reduce the amount of mucus that builds up, which, I believe, worsens the condition.

▷ The next point is especially important, breathe through your nose as this will help moisten the air, making life so much easier for your lungs. This is especially true in winter, when the air is cold, but should be done even during the summer. When you are not exercising, try breathing through your nose as it will make a huge difference to your asthma.

Massage

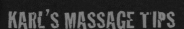

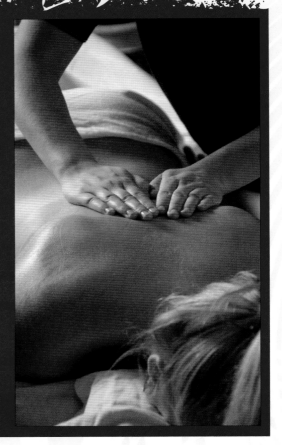

KARL'S MASSAGE TIPS

Am I supposed to take off my underwear when I get a massage?

Many people prefer to keep their underwear on during a massage, while others prefer to be completely nude. It's totally up to you.

If your problem areas are your lower back, hips, buttocks or groin, tight-fitting underwear can sometimes get in the way of massage work and going nude might just be the best option. Either way, you will be fully covered at all times with towels so don't worry!

What if the massage is too light?

Tell your masseur! There is nothing worse than lying there with no pressure being applied. If it is still too light after you have said something, then cancel the massage, because you are getting very few benefits from it bar some stress release.

For many people, massage may seem to be too much of a luxury to have, or is only thought of when they have an injury and want to try loosen it out. Massage has so many benefits, from de-stressing to weight loss. Regular massage can help to break down fat, improve metabolism and help digestion. If your muscles are sore, a good deep tissue massage can help to loosen out all those aches and pains. Let's look at the different types of massage and how they can help you.

Ki-Massage

This was developed in Ireland by the Irish Health Culture Association (IHCA) which, today, is one of the leading training organisations. The IHCA ensures the therapists it trains have gone through a very strict training programme before it considers them qualified.

In Ki-Massage, you can experience a feeling of deep relaxation, which enables you to withdraw from everyday stress and come back to face life with new energy. This has an extraordinary effect on your health and mental well being and, when repeated over a period of time, brings about a positive outlook that can help you to cope more easily with what is happening in your life. It is both relaxing and invigorating and stimulates circulation in a natural way and helps to stop you becoming up-tight.

Sports

Sports massage was designed for athletes, but is useful for anyone with chronic pain, injury or range-of-motion issues.

Sports massage was originally developed to help athletes prepare their bodies for optimal performance, recover after a big event or function well during training. Sports massage emphasises prevention and healing of injuries to the muscles and tendons.

Thai massage

Thai massage can only be described as a combination of massage and yoga. The masseur will use his/her feet and arms to bend your body into different positions, generally based on the pressure points of the body. It is a very different type of massage and has many benefits from my experience such as improved flexibility. You will be sore the day after the massage but 2 days later you will feel like a new person. It is a totally different feeling from any other type of massage, tougher and firmer but with great physical benefits.

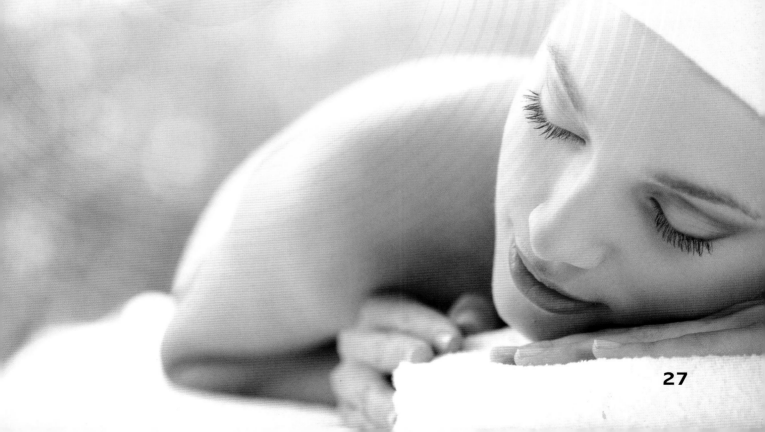

Reflexology

Reflexology is based on the theory that each body part is represented on the hands and feet and that pressing on specific areas on the hands or feet can have therapeutic effects in other parts of the body. A reflexologist focuses mainly on your feet and it can relieve stress and promote relaxation. Reflexology can also improve circulation, reduce pain, soothe tired feet and encourage overall healing.

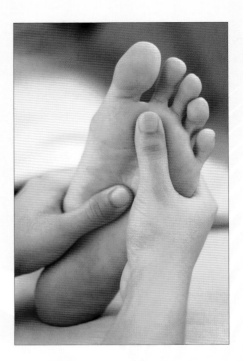

Benefits of massage

A weekly massage will have great benefits to your health. Below is a list of the benefits of massage:

- Increases blood supply to your joints.
- Produces muscular relaxation.
- Prevents muscle tears or strains by keeping your muscles limber.
- Attracts blood from internal parts.
- Stimulates and soothes nerves.
- Improves the body's ability to use nutrients.
- Removes effluent matter or waste more quickly.
- Helps remove cellulite.

Massage gets the healing energy flowing in the body as a whole as well as in the sick or injured part. This is particularly beneficial to elderly people, and for those who are sick or are incapacitated. Everyone can benefit from massage, there are areas of sluggish circulation not effected by exercise, which massage will benefit directly. A good masseur or masseuse must develop the ability to relax themselves completely – to absorb him or herself in the work to bring about a proper state of relaxation in the client. On having a massage, you would see why this ability of the masseur has been traditionally held in high regard.

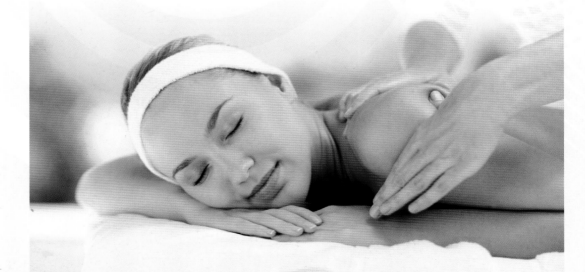

Let's get going

If you want to change, join me and learn from me, I will show you the way! Have you had enough of being permanently tired, depressed and not fitting into any of your clothes? Are you ready to change your life for good and improve the lives of those around you?

There are three steps to getting you on the road to a healthy, revitalised you. Let's get started.

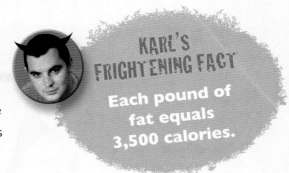

KARL'S FRIGHTENING FACT

Each pound of fat equals 3,500 calories.

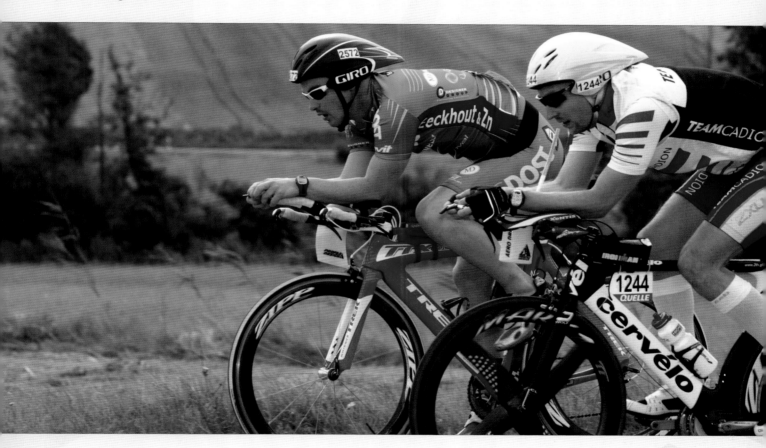

STEP 1 Body types

Which body type are you? Why is your body type important? Well I feel that it's essential for you to be able to identify what body type you are before you start training. This is your starting point towards being an educated fitness consumer. The good news is that all body types can achieve fantastic results – if you are trying to gain weight even with the fastest metabolism it can be done, similarly, if you're an endomorph, then it is possible to lose weight – the even better news is that I am going to show you how.

Men and women have different concerns when it comes to their body types. First, I am going to look at the male body type – OK guys, listen up, read the three different body types below and see which one you are.

Men

Endomorph
(the John Hayes)

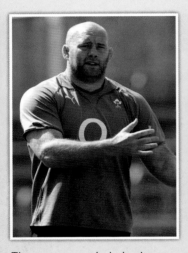

The more rounded physique that is prone to very easy weight gain, your food intake might be less than other people but you find you put weight on really easily. This is normally due to a very slow metabolism. It is a great physique for strength and power, but it can be extremely frustrating when trying to lose weight!

High-protein diets will tend to bulk you up, so low GI plans will be more beneficial for you.

Ectomorph
(the Peter Crouch)

The super skinny person that has found it very hard to put on weight all of his life no matter what he does or eats. This is normally due to an extremely fast metabolism. I know this may sound amazing but, trust me, it can be equally frustrating as ectomorphs find it incredibly hard to gain weight and to gain muscle. The way forward is to eat meals every 2 to 3 hours and eat protein with every meal, this combined with an exercise plan will reap great rewards, though it will take some time depending on just how fast your metabolism is. I have a client who gained 2 stones over the course of a year and a half and has to work hard to keep it there.

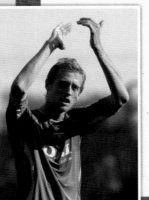

Mesomorph
(the George Clooney)

A combination of both endomorph and ectomorph, this body type finds it easy to lose weight and easy to gain strength and muscle. Their metabolism is generally high and, when your food is good, then the weight will decrease very fast. While you may put on weight quickly, you can lose it just as fast!

Mesomorphs need intense workouts to get the most from their muscle tone, lower their body fat and emphasise their shape. Adding an extra portion of protein into your diet can do wonders for reducing your body fat and helping to get the tone that you always wanted.

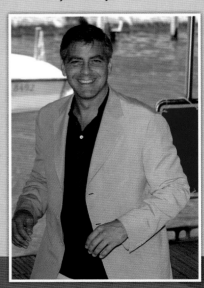

Women

With the men aware of their closest body type, now it's time for all you women to find which body shape you are. There are so many different varieties used in the fitness/diet industry, so I have simplified it down to just four. Excited? Well, see which shape you are.

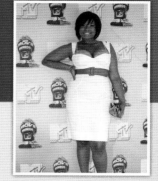

Celery (the Keira Knightley)

You have a slim body with hips and shoulders that are roughly the same width. You often find it hard to maintain your weight and generally can eat whatever you like as your metabolism is fast. Many people think that this is an enviable shape to have, but it is equally frustrating for those who struggle to put on weight. If this is a physique that you have, try plenty of body resistance exercises, such as press-ups, squats and lunges.

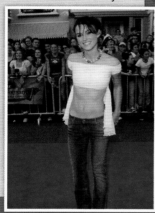

Apple (the Jennifer Hudson)

This is one of the more typical Irish body shapes. You carry all your weight around your mid-section from your chest to your pelvis, often with slim legs and arms. You've found that as you got older, you developed a muffin top, that turned into a spare tyre that is now hard to shift. As your metabolism slows down, your body develops fat around the mid-section. Also known as the 'wine wobble', this weight comes from food/alcohol and can be very stubborn. If this body type describes you, aim to do plenty of interval training combined with fast, light weights with high reps and an improved diet.

Pear (the Jennifer Lopez)

You have a body that is prone to weight gain, your hips are wider than your shoulders, and you have lots of curves for good measure. You find it hard to lose fat and when you tried weights before, you thought that you built muscle very quickly. The best workouts for this body shape require lots of intervals combined with light weight workouts, featuring exercises such as side leg raises, bum kicks and pelvic floor kicks, these are great for you, obviously combined with a good diet.

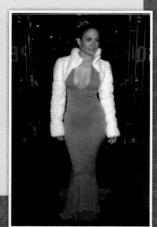

Hour Glass (the Marilyn Monroe)

The typical 1950s screen siren look with broad shoulders, a narrow waist and curvaceous hips. Your weight can go up or down depending on your diet and, when you knuckle down, you can get in great shape very easily. This is one of the more enviable body shapes. It's sexy, feminine and, despite the press coverage, the body shape that most women want! Your metabolism is consistent and when you improve your diet, your weight/shape returns very quickly.

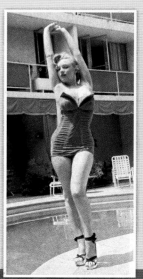

STEP 2 Measuring your progress

Have you found which body type you are? Now that you know that, let's look at how you can measure your progress during the coming weeks and months.

From all my experience with my clients, I find that it is essential to set goals and measure progress on a weekly basis. This is short-term goal setting at its best, we will look at goal setting later in the book in Section 4.

There are several different ways to track your progress and I am going to give you all the information your need to make up your own mind about what suits you best.

Body Mass Index (BMI)

BMI is the current standard for measuring people that is used across the world. Yet, myself – and many other fitness experts – aren't fans of it. Put basically it says that if you are a certain height, then you should be a certain weight. The formula for getting your BMI is your weight in kilograms divided by your height in metres squared.

The reason I don't use this measurement is that it doesn't take into account your body type or bone structure – and different body types have different bone structures.

There are several different classifications: under 18.5 is classified as underweight, 18.5 to 24.5 is classified as normal weight, 25 to 29.5 is classified as being overweight, 30 and above is classified as being obese, and 40 and above is classified as morbidly obese.

Body fat

Body fat is measured using callipers or body fat sensors and is a far more accurate way of giving you feedback. If using the callipers, you pinch the body at three distinct areas: your shoulder blade, your tricep and your pelvis. While there is an element of unreliability, it is usually a quite accurate method.

If you are using the sensors, then place you hands or your feet on pads. These pads send a signal though your body via bio impedance and give your results on the screen. To be honest, unless you are using an expensive piece of equipment, these are generally very unreliable and can give you different results each time.

KARL'S FRIGHT'ENING FACT

Around the week of your period you will be between 3-5 pounds heavier due to water retention.

Inches

This is my personal favourite. Sometimes weight will be slow to come off, but your inches will reduce quickly. Simply buy a measuring tape and your good to go. There are seven points on the body that I measure: neck, right bicep, chest (across the nipple line), waist (across the belly button), hips (across the hip bones), right leg (halfway between the knee and hip) and your calf. I find using a tape measure the most effective way to see progress as its reliable and covers all the body areas. You can track your progress easily and cheaply too.

Scales

Another great way to measure your progress. Though there are a few points to note.

▸ Buy yourself a good set of scales, either an old-school Seca doctors scales or if you want to buy digital, I would recommend spending between €70 and €100. Again, the cheaper digital models tend not to be as accurate, making you more frustrated! Some scales offer silver pads with bio impedance, giving you your BMI and body fat. Unfortunately, many of these don't work, giving you different reading each time. I would recommend a normal set of scales to measure your weight only.

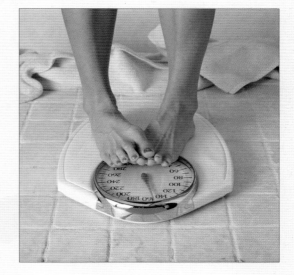

▸ Ensure the scales are on a level floor, tiles are better than wooden floors.

▸ Always weigh yourself first thing in the morning as this is your real weight. You will always be heavier in the evening, sometimes by as much as 5 pounds.

▸ Weigh yourself once per week.

▸ Aim to weigh yourself at the same time each week.

STEP 3   Measuring your fitness level

There are three tests that I am going to show you that will measure your fitness levels. They are so simple to do and will give you an accurate, quick gauge of how fit you are as well as giving you another way to measure your progress in future. The only thing you will need is a clock, it's that simple! Ideally, try to do all three tests in the same session. Take a 4-minute break between each test to enable your heart rate to settle back to a normal level.

Test 1: Aerobic endurance

You will need a 12-inch high bench, or the bottom stair in your home will do just fine. You are going to step on and off for 3 minutes. Try to hold a steady pace all the way through. There is a piece of equipment called a metronome that you can use to help you keep a steady rhythm, but if you don't have one of these, saying, 'Up, up, down, down', will help you. Immediately after the 3 minutes, take your pulse. Using either two fingers placed at the side of your neck, or at the base of your wrist, then just time it for a minute on the clock. Compare your results in the chart below.

3-Minute Step Test (Men) - Heart Rate

Age	18-25	26-35	36-45	46-55	56-65	65+
Excellent	<79	<81	<83	<87	<86	<88
Good	79-89	81-89	83-96	87-97	86-97	88-96
Above Average	90-99	90-99	97-103	98-105	98-103	97-103
Average	100-105	100-107	104-112	106-116	104-112	104-113
Below Average	106-116	108-117	113-119	117-122	113-120	114-120
Poor	117-128	118-128	120-130	123-132	121-129	121-130
Very Poor	>128	>128	>130	>132	>129	>130

3-Minute Step Test (Women) - Heart Rate

Age	18-25	26-35	36-45	46-55	56-65	65+
Excellent	<85	<88	<90	<94	<95	<90
Good	85-98	88-99	90-102	94-104	95-104	90-102
Above Average	99-108	100-111	103-110	105-115	105-112	103-115
Average	109-117	112-119	111-118	116-120	113-118	116-122
Below Average	118-126	120-126	119-128	121-129	119-128	123-128
Poor	127-140	127-138	129-140	130-135	129-139	129-134
Very Poor	>140	>138	>140	>135	>139	>134

Test 2: Testing abdominal strength

How did the step up test go? Well, this test is even simpler. Lie on your back on the floor with your knees bent. Place your hands on your thighs and, as you sit up, squeeze your stomach. Come up high enough for your hands to touch your knees. It's important not to pull your neck up, keep your eyes looking towards the ceiling, head totally relaxed. I see people all the time who use their hands to drag their neck, all you're doing here is damaging your neck I'm afraid. If you get any neck pain at all, be sure to stop straight away. Do as many sit-ups as you can in 1 minute and compare with the chart below for your results.

1-Minute Sit-Up Test (Men)

Age	18-25	26-35	36-45	46-55	56-65	65+
Excellent	>49	>45	>41	>35	>31	>28
Good	44-49	40-45	35-41	29-35	25-31	22-28
Above Average	39-43	35-39	30-34	25-28	21-24	19-21
Average	35-38	31-34	27-29	22-24	17-20	15-18
Below Average	31-34	29-30	23-26	18-21	13-16	11-14
Poor	25-30	22-28	17-22	13-17	9-12	7-10
Very Poor	<25	<22	<17	<9	<9	<7

1-Minute Sit-Up Test (Women)

Age	18-25	26-35	36-45	46-55	56-65	65+
Excellent	>43	>39	>33	>27	>24	>23
Good	37-43	33-39	27-33	22-27	18-24	17-23
Above Average	33-36	29-32	23-26	18-21	13-17	14-16
Average	29-32	25-28	19-22	14-17	10-12	11-13
Below Average	25-28	21-24	15-18	10-13	7-9	5-10
Poor	18-24	13-20	7-14	5-9	3-6	2-4
Very Poor	<18	<20	<7	<5	<3	<2

Test 3: Testing your upper body strength

For this test, we use the age-old press-up test. Ideally, try to do the military style press-up, with a nice straight back, chest to the floor and straight back. If you find that you can't do this, then try the less strenuous version and place your knees on the floor, shoulder-width apart. If you are doing this version, ensure to have your hips parallel with your knees, as most people have their bum too high. Do as many as you can — until there is no more strength in your arms — for 1 minute. Then, check your progress with the chart below.

Push-Up Test (Men)

Age	17-19	20-29	30-39	40-49	50-59	60-65
Excellent	> 56	> 47	> 41	> 34	> 31	> 30
Good	47-56	39-47	34-41	28-34	25-31	24-30
Above Average	35-46	30-39	25-33	21-28	18-24	17-23
Average	19-34	17-29	13-24	11-20	9-17	6-16
Below Average	11-18	10-16	8-12	6-10	5-8	3-5
Poor	4-10	4-9	2-7	1-5	1-4	1-2
Very Poor	< 4	< 4	< 2	0	0	0

Push-Up Test (Women)

Age	17-19	20-29	30-39	40-49	50-59	60-65
Excellent	> 35	> 36	> 37	> 31	> 25	> 23
Good	27-35	30-36	30-37	25-31	21-25	19-23
Above Average	21-27	23-29	22-30	18-24	15-20	13-18
Average	11-20	12-22	10-21	8-17	7-14	5-12
Below Average	6-10	7-11	5-9	4-7	3-6	2-4
Poor	2-5	2-6	1-4	1-3	1-2	1
Very Poor	0-1	0-1	0	0	0	0

These three tests will give you a great idea about how fit (or unfit) you are. Regardless of your results, this is your starting point. We all need one, it just provides a great way for you to measure your progress, re-test yourself after 4 weeks and you will be amazed by the results.

At this point you have all the basics. You have now found your body type, decided how you are going to measure your progress and also measured your fitness levels. You are good to get started in to the programme that will change the rest of your life.

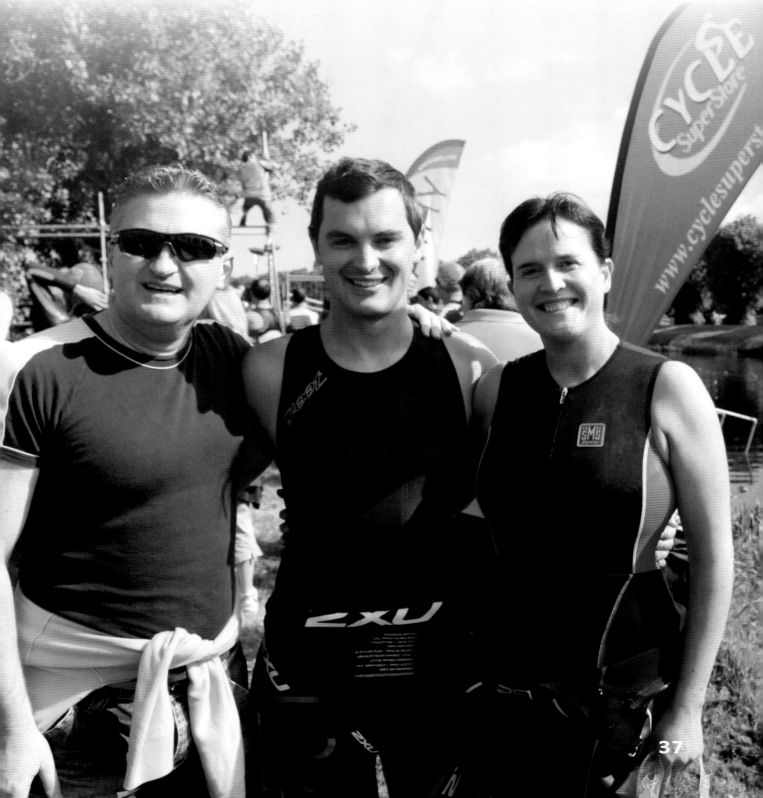

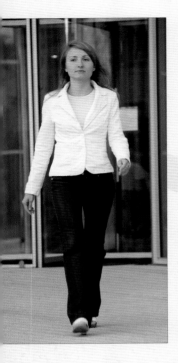

Health screening questionnaire

Before you start you plan, I want you to assess your health. Take 2 minutes to fill out the form below. This is an essential component, ensuring that you are fit to start training straight away, if you have answered yes to any of the questions, then always ensure that you get your GP's approval before you start any exercise plan.

Remember, Rome wasn't built in a day, it's essential to have a clean bill of health before starting your training, a healthy foundation leads to a healthy body.

Health history and screening

Do you have now, or have you had in the past, any of the following conditions? (Please tick your answer.)

1 History of heart problems, chest pain or stroke?

Yes   No

2 Elevated or low blood pressure?

Yes   No

3 Any chronic illness or conditions?

Yes   No

4 Advice from a doctor not to exercise?

Yes   No

5 Recent surgery (past 12 months)?

Yes   No

6 Pregnancy (currently or within three months)?

Yes   No

7 Asthma or history of breathing or lung problems?

Yes   No

8 Muscle, joint or back disorder or any previous injury still affecting you?

Yes   No

9 Diabetes or a thyroid condition?

Yes   No

10 Smoking habit?

Yes   No

11 Obesity (more than 20 per cent over your ideal body weight)?

Yes   No

12 Increased blood cholesterol?

Yes   No

13 History of heart problems in your immediate family?

Yes   No

14 Hernia or any condition that may be aggravated by resistance/weight training?

Yes   No

15 Osteoporosis or other bone-density problems?

Yes   No

16 Difficulty with physical exercise?

Yes   No

17 Are you taking any prescribed medication or drugs? If yes, please list the medication the reason and dose. If necessary, discuss this with your GP.

Measurements sheet

This sheet is to help you track your progress over a six-week period. Measure your body parts on week 1 and then measure the same day every week to see just how you are getting on, write it down for further motivation. I find that using this sheet every 2 weeks is one of the best ways to track your progress, as you see the inches coming off your body. Simply get the measuring tape out and measure all the body parts listed on the sheet, write down the measurements and every 2 weeks do it again. If you can't do it yourself, then get someone to help you out!

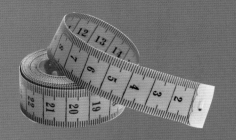

	Week 1	Week 2	Week 3	Week 4	Week 5	Week 6
Weight						
Neck						
Right arm						
Chest						
Waist						
Hips						
Right leg						

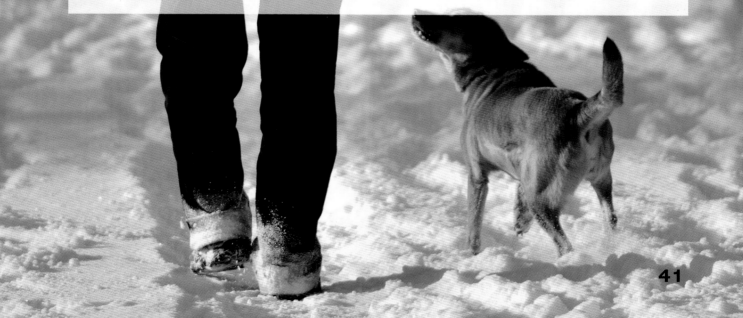

I first met Karl in 1996 at my nephew's birthday party. Six years later, when I was fifty-five, I realised I needed help if I was to achieve any level of fitness. I turned to Karl who had just started his career as training instructor. For the next eight years he guided me on a course of exercises, stretches and modest weights and has helped me achieve a level of fitness that has enhanced every area of my life.

My singing and breathing have benefited greatly. I have come to realise that even a moderate level of fitness improves my ability to sing and play an instrument for two hours on stage. I am sixty-five now and I try to exercise every day. I have found it very helpful to keep a log of what I do. This means that I have a target to achieve each week. On average, I will walk twenty miles a week, do stretching exercises four times and weights twice. I always look forward to the severe stretching with which Karl finishes our weekly session. This can verge on painful but always releases something into the system which provides a natural high. The weights are my least favourite form of exercise but I only have eight different routines so I get them done fairly quickly.

I still struggle with my weight as I am partial to the spuds. Karl has tried to help me in this area too. Today, my work takes me to Bath in England. I am here to play at the Glastonbury Festival where I will perform for ninety minutes in front of 10,000 people in a very hot marquee at ten o'clock on Saturday night. It requires an element of fitness to perform at this level. This morning I did twenty minutes stretching in my hotel room followed by a five-mile walk down by the banks of the old canal. I also do leg exercises each day to aid my ageing knees which suffered damage in the 1960s when I was a 'pint of Guinness' prop forward. I have been on the road for forty-five years now. This exercise routine, which has become part of my life, enables me to continue doing what I love to do. I would urge everyone, young and old, to get involved … it's never too late to start … 'Ride On'

'The greatest
wealth is health.'

Virgil

Nutrition

The time for quick-fix diets is over. In these pages, you won't find a high-protein or high-fat diet that you can't keep up, and there are no special shakes or bars. You will find the real solution to health and well being, the real weight-loss solution and the real way to keep the weight off. To view our many recommended recipes, simply visit *www.henryfitnesscentre.com*.

Before we get into more detail, let's take a look at all those scary words that are talked about so much that confuse you when it comes to nutrition.

Words you need to know

Calories

A calorie is simply a unit of energy — it tells you how much energy there is in a food. The government have stated that both men and women should consume 2,000 calories a day from our diet. This has increased for women over the past few years from 1,500 (it has always been 2,000 for men). As the nation's waistlines expand, the government is merely expanding our calorie intake guidelines, rather than tackling the problem itself. In my opinion, I feel that the old guideline of 1,500 calories for women and 2,000 for men is far more appropriate.

The real view of calorie intake depends on your day. If you spend all day sitting, then obviously you need fewer calories than if you are moving.

Protein

Protein has two main functions in a diet: growth and repair. Without enough protein in your diet, you will take longer to recover from your workouts and you will have less muscle tone in your body. Some fitness professionals recommend protein shakes to get extra protein into a diet, but I feel that this is totally unnecessary unless you have a deficiency in your diet, aim to get as much of your protein from natural foods as possible. Foods high in protein also tend to be high in iron and B vitamins too.

So how much protein should you take in a day? If you are working out on a regular basis, you will need roughly 1.2 to 1.4 grams per kilo of body weight — so if you weigh 70 kg, then you should be eating 84 grams of protein per day. Don't get too caught up in the numbers, simply aim to eat a piece of protein with your lunch and one with your dinner, and you will be fine.

Karl's real results food plan will:

▷ Give you more energy.
▷ Improve your skin.
▷ Improve your mood.
▷ Increase your metabolism.
▷ Help you lose weight safely and slowly.

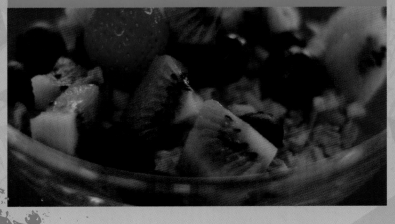

Reasons diets don't work

Low energy
No exercise
Radical changes
Lack of motivation
No lifestyle change
Emotional eating
Food cravings
No support

Carbohydrates

Carbohydrates give you energy! Lower your carbohydrate intake and you will have less energy for sure. As you will see below, not all carbohydrates are the same. Carbohydrates are also high in fibre, B vitamins and minerals too.

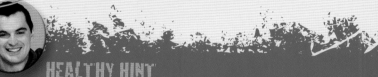

HEALTHY HINT

Carbohydrates are actually good for you! They provide the energy in your diet, cutting out carbs is the same as putting no fuel in the car! The important element is the type of carbohydrate that you eat.

There are two main types of carbohydrates: white and brown. White carbs are full of starch and are lower in nutrients. They lead to bloating and are ingrained into the Irish diet. Brown carbohydrates are full of fibre and lead to a more consistent energy stream. They are full of goodness.

Type of carbohydrate	Effect on body	Nutrition value
White	Bloating, energy sapping	Low
Brown	Sustained energy	Full of fibre

In summary, the big four you should change are:

Change from	Change to
White bread	Brown bread
White pasta	Brown pasta
White rice	Brown rice
Potatoes	Sweet potatoes

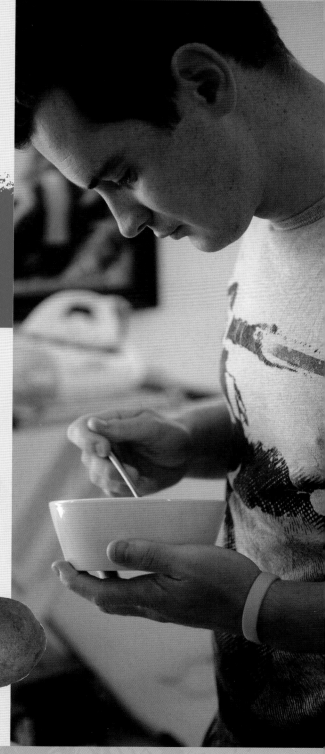

Fat

Fats are often confused as being a bad part of a diet. Yet they are essential for health and for your immune system to function properly.

There are two main types of fat: saturated and unsaturated. The unsaturated fats are the good ones, they even help you to lower your cholesterol and your risk of heart disease. They can even help you get leaner! Let's take a look at fats in more detail.

The table below tells you all about fats – it really is that basic.

KARL'S FRIGHTENING FACT

Low-fat or fat-free products are often far worse than the original version of the product! The original nutrients are taken out and replaced with artificial colours and preservatives that are often far less healthy than the original! So steer well clear of them!

Type of fat	Sources	Information	Example
Saturated	Animal fats, palm oil	▶ Increase cholesterol and risk of heart disease ▶ No benefits to body	Fatty meats, any product with palm oil, full-fat dairy products
Unsaturated	Nuts, oils	▶ Essential for the body	Nuts (unsalted), olive oil
Trans fats	Hydrogenated fats	▶ The most dangerous	Cereal bars, pastries, cakes, biscuits

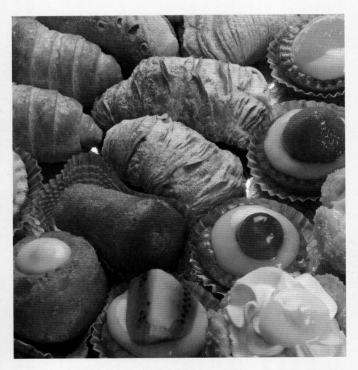

When reading labels, looking out for palm oil and you will be amazed at just how many foods contain it! As you can see, some fats are essential for our diet, so don't cut them out!

The final type of fat mentioned that I want to talk to you about are trans fats.

These are the most harmful and most dangerous kind of fat. They are manufactured when liquid fats are converted into hard fats. They increase the levels of bad cholesterol and reduce the levels of good cholesterol in your body, rapidly increasing your levels of cardiovascular disease. Can you guess what they are contained in? Pastries, pies and tarts, many low-fat products, cakes and bakery products.

Vitamins and minerals

Vitamins are essential for the immune system, as they help the brain function properly and play an important role in converting your food into energy as well as ensuring you have healthy skin, hair and nails.

Slightly different from vitamins, minerals are essential for body functions, such as nerve function, cell growth and muscle/nerve function.

The whole area of vitamins and minerals can be very confusing, so let's take a look at the table below where I will make everything easy for you to understand.

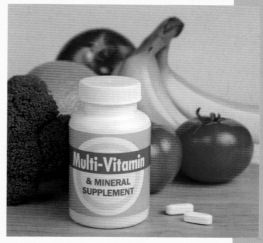

Vitamin/mineral	What it does	Food source	How much?
Vitamin A	▸ Vision ▸ Skin	Fish, eggs, butter, cheese	700 mg men, 600 mg women
Vitamin C	▸ Healthy bones, teeth ▸ Blood vessels ▸ Iron absorption ▸ Immune system	Fruit, vegetables	40 mg men and women
Vitamin E	▸ Full of antioxidants ▸ Reduces post-muscle soreness	Fish, eggs, butter, nuts	10 mg men and women
Calcium	▸ Healthy bones, teeth ▸ Nerve function	Milk and dairy products, green leafy vegetables	1,000 mg men, 700 mg women
Iron	▸ Prevents anaemia ▸ Helps the formation of red blood cells	Meat, wholegrain cereals, pulses, spinach, cabbage	8.7 mg men, 14.8 mg women
Magnesium	▸ Bones ▸ Nerve function ▸ Cell formation	Cereals, fruit, vegetables	300 mg men, 270 mg women
Potassium	▸ Muscle/nerve function	Fruit, cereals, vegetables	3,500 mg men and women
Zinc	▸ Immune system ▸ Skin ▸ Cell growth	Wholegrain cereals, meat, milk, dairy products	9.5 mg men, 7.0 mg women

Many people recommend supplements for your diet, but I am always slow to recommend supplements unless you have a deficiency in your diet. As a vegetarian myself, sometimes I take supplements when I feel that my diet isn't delivering all the nutrients I need.

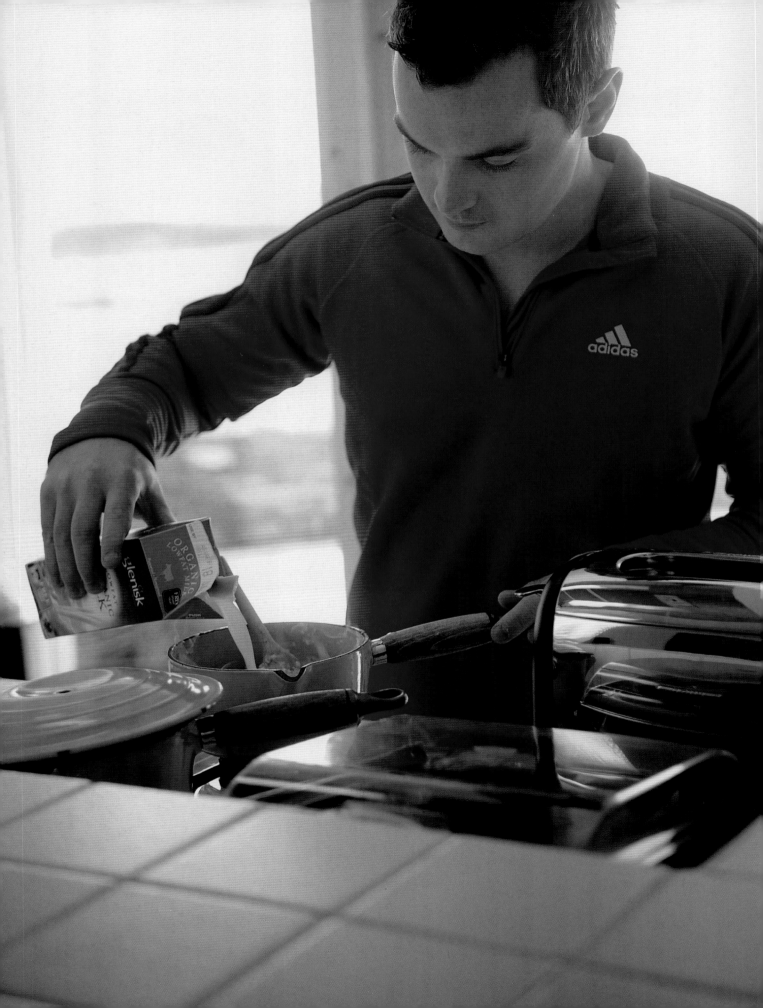

The big mineral for women is obviously iron. Around your time of the month, a lot of iron can be lost and this leads to anaemia. I certainly think that an iron supplement may be useful for women. When you look at your diet, you will know straight away if you are getting all the nutrients you need into it. A multivitamin will be perfect to give you all the nutrients that you need if you find that you aren't getting them from your diet. In an ideal world, you would get everything you need from your food intake, but as is often the case with our busy lives, we don't get everything we need this way, if this is the case then a good multivitamin will help. Bio-Strath is my favourite, it's old school, full of nutrients and available nationwide.

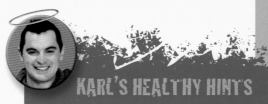

KARL'S HEALTHY HINTS

Why whole grains are better:

▷ No cholesterol
▷ Low in fat
▷ Soluble/insoluble
▷ Digest slower/feel fuller longer
▷ Low GI (see p.57)

I have thrown a lot information at you, so let's take a break for a second and absorb all the information.

Below is a chart that simplifies things even more for you.

Nutrient	Food	Function
Protein	Meat, fish, eggs	Repair and growth
Carbohydrates	Brown pasta, brown bread	Energy
Fats	Oils	Skin, hair, nails
Vitamins	Fruit and vegetables	Body functions
Minerals	Fruit and vegetables	Body functions
Fibre	Wholegrain foods	Digestion/bowel

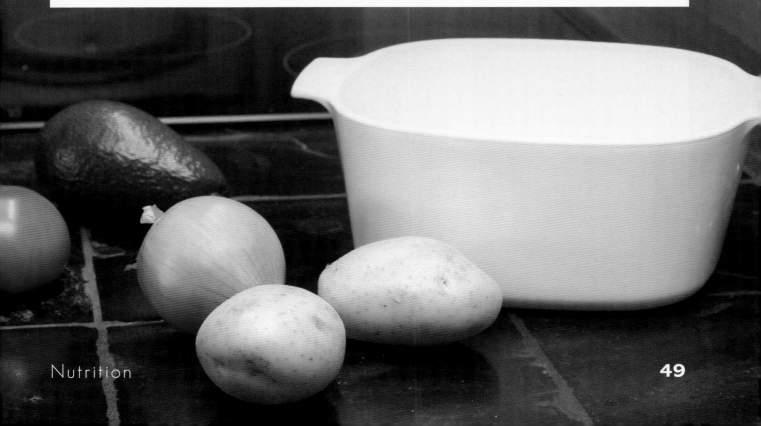

'Would the big girl at the back please move forward.' That would have meant me, approximately three years ago.

Now, it's, 'Would the Olympic Triathlete please stand up.'

Yes, that's me on my feet! Me – Ellen. Would you believe it? I can hardly believe it myself sometimes, but it is true and one of my greatest achievements to date, and one of my personal proudest moments, was when I reached my goal. How did I go from that girl at the back, to this triathlete? Well, with a lot of hard work, focus, determination, sacrifice and fabulous fun.

I remember taking my first steps into the gym, having had an initial chat with Karl. I desperately wanted to make a change. I no longer wanted to be 'the big girl', the girl floating around in the 'cover-up tent outfits'. I wanted to find the real me under all the layers and unleash the hidden athlete.

Karl and I started working together in the gym and I went through the dreaded 'step onto the scales, Ellen'. I just had to accept where I was and focus on where I wanted to go. I will never forget the initial body measurements. Oh my God! The horror! How had I let this happen? Well, to put it simply, by eating all the wrong foods and, of course, a complete lack of continual and consistent exercise.

Bust size, *That's impossible.*

Waist size, *Not even conceivable.*

Leg measurements, *Only a sumo wrestler should have legs that size.*

Arm measurements, *Ellen, have you had a secret career in arm wrestling?*

Neck measurement, *What?*

All my own thoughts about the results.

Karl simply wrote them down and calmly assured me that, if I worked hard with him, there was an Elle McPherson hidden away! Elle, the beautiful BOD, never materialised but, as I worked hard in the gym, gradually the inches came off every part of my body.

I am a person that needs a goal and Karl quickly cottoned on to this. The goal could be the unworn 'cute jeans' that I couldn't hammer myself into or, the forthcoming event or wedding I was attending. Gradually, he would sow the seeds for our next goal. I will never forget the day he suggested that we would go out for a run on our next session.

What? Me running? 'I'll give it a go,' I said. 'What have I got to lose?"

Karl set the stopwatch and simply said, 'Just run for as long as you can.'

Off I started with Karl running alongside me. He had lots of words of encouragement for me and reminded me to breathe. Breathing properly is helpful but, believe me, it is easier said than done.

Karl has a little technique to keep you going. He places a finger gently in the base of your back, which projects you forward. I suddenly thought, *I'm off. This is cool, I've cracked this running lark.*

He said, 'Keep going, Ellen. Keep going.' I finally stopped when I thought my heart would burst out of my chest and I would expire. I leaned over, gasping for breath, hands on my knees and Karl stopped the watch. 'Well done, Ellen. You did very well.'

'Thanks, Karl, that was great. How did I do?'

'Well, Ellen, you ran for exactly three minutes.'

'Three minutes! Three minutes?'

I realised I had a long road ahead but, it was a start, albeit a small start.

Six months later, I travelled to Connemara to compete in the half-marathon. My friends and family came to cheer me on and support me. I ran for all I was worth and, when I crossed the line, I felt so damn great. What a transformation.

Then I was wondering, *What's next?* A Triathlon, that's what's next!

I hadn't been on a bike since I was a teenager and the same with the swimming. Baby steps, one step at a time, a slow build up. Suddenly, things start to feel easier, more natural and then, one day, you know, 'I can do this. This is a strong possibility.' Karl kept me strong, focused and kept the encouragement alive. I hooked up with my good friend Maurice and my sister Niamh and we started training together. No more late nights and no vino on Saturday night. An early-to-bed and early-start-on-the-roads every Sunday morning. Not easy when it's dark, cold and often raining. We kept the momentum going and set a regular training programme in place. 'No slackers need apply' was our motto.

We had good sessions, hard training and, of course, each of us had our off days, but we propped one another up and, without fail, despite bad conditions or feeling low, we kept going.

We had such a laugh together. Whatever training we were doing and would usually go for breakfast, lunch or a coffee afterwards, to discuss tactics and find out how each of us felt.

I recall a memorable session on the bikes in the Phoenix Park, when we were continually pelted in the face with driving rain and, for the last few kilometres, just to bring us home, we had hailstones bombarding us. At that stage, I was too into it and knew there was nothing going to stop me. I was going to do this.

TriAthy race day in Athy, County Kildare. Again, a great posse of friends and family were on board to cheer me on, slagging me with, 'Ellen, for God's sake don't get dragged out of the river.'

All good fun but they know how much their presence meant to me.

Countdown, 'Five, four, three, two, one. Go!'

I'm in the river getting kicked, punched, wild splashing and, after about thirty seconds, I'm out on my own and off.

'Keep going, keep going, keep breathing,' I was saying to myself and, suddenly, I'm out of the river and running towards Transition 1, pulling off the wet suit at high speed and getting on the bike.

Karl is shouting, 'Great swim, Ellen. Well done, keep going.'

'Eye of the Tiger' music playing in my head. Ha, Ha! Onto the bike, in the tri-suit (not the most flattering attire but what the hell). I would not have contemplated getting into a suit like that a year or so ago.

I'm feeling good and peddling for all I'm worth out on the bike course, wind in my face. Phase 2 is underway.

It was so amazing to witness some of the professionals and elite athletes whizzing past but, again, I'm here, competing and focused. 'Keep the legs moving, Ellen. Keep going,' I remember telling myself.

Into Transition 3. Quick change and out on the run.

Now, I'm really enjoying myself, 'I'm nearly home, two-thirds down just one part left to go. Keep drinking the water, the legs pumping and take it all in. This is great.'

Soon, the finish line is in sight and I can hear the roars of encouragement from my gang, 'Go, Ellen, go.'

As I ran on, one of them shouted at me. 'Ellen, how do you feel? How was it?'

I remember breaking my heart laughing and shouting back, 'It was just a walk in the park!'

As I crossed the finish line, with my arms punching the air, I could stand up and say to myself, 'Ellen, you are no longer that person 'at the back', you are now an Olympic Triathlete.'

Being fit, healthy and in better shape is unquestionably the best feeling in the world. I feel better, stronger, younger. I eat much better. I am more able to cope with all that life throws at me and, best of all, I can get into those 'cute jeans'.

Quick-fix diets

Every quick-fix solution on the market comes with the obligatory diet that starves your body of essential nutrients and reduces your energy levels. Generally, within 6 weeks, you have all but given up on the diet, reintroducing foods that you swore you would never eat again.

These diets work off either one of two principles. First, you reduce your calorific intake and spend the whole day counting the calories and analysing every single food label for the calories that are in them. The second principle is cutting out one essential nutrient of your diet. You either cut out protein, carbohydrates or fat, reduction of one of these nutrients generally leads to weight loss and, generally, it is carbohydrates that are eliminated. But, guess what? When you go back to normal eating, you put the weight back on – and very often you put even more on!

These crash diets are short term, they will never last. I'm sure you have seen it with your friends and maybe even yourself, every year the same thing happens.

The time for these quick fixes is over! I am going to show you how to eat normally, have that pizza that you love so much and create balance in your diet that will lead to weight loss and maintaining your goal weight. I love restaurants and eating out and why should you have to give this up? The simple answer is, you shouldn't!

Karl's 4 reasons quick-fix diets don't work

▷ Your body isn't getting all the nutrients it needs.

▷ Your metabolism slows down.

▷ You cut everything out, swearing never to touch them again.

▷ It's impossible to maintain for life.

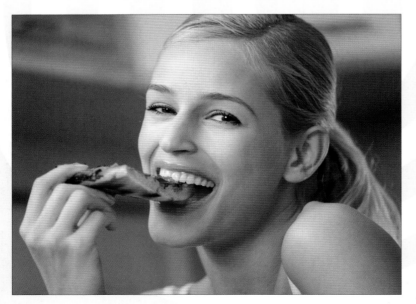

Have you had enough of the quick-fix diets, restricting the vital nutrients your body needs and starving yourself for weeks on end? Would you like to lose weight for life, easily and steadily? How about being able to have your Chinese or pizza and still lose weight? Sound too good to be true? The good news is that it can be done and I am going to show you how.

First, let's look at some of the quick-fix diets on the market and what they are all about.

Atkins

The Atkins diet was probably the biggest and most successful diet of the past 20 years! It worked off a very simple principle, high protein and no carbohydrates. By eliminating carbs from your diet, you are forcing your body into what is call ketosis – what this means is that your body eats itself and its own fat stores. While you will lose weight initially, in the longer run, you will develop the infamous ketosis breath, hard skin and cold sores. Experts expect other ailments to show themselves as a result of this diet but as there have been no long-term studies of a high-protein diet, there is no consensus on what these might be.

Karl's little experiment

The next time you are in the supermarket play the trolley game. Look at that trolley that has been left stranded and try to match it to the person who comes to pick it up. You will find this: a trolley full of sugar-fuelled, non-nutritious junk food will be matched by a person who is unhealthy and overweight, possibly even a family that is overweight. Am I wrong? Try it for yourself!

The Atkins diet doesn't last long term because you need carbohydrates for energy and health. I have recently read some trainers discussing the fact that you don't need carbohydrates for energy and that protein is sufficient to meet all your energy requirements. Not in my opinion. If I cut out carbohydrates, I get tired more easily, simple as that. I can't function, concentrate or work even half of my day. Carbohydrates are essential for health and energy, cut them out at your peril. Try it for yourself and see what you think.

Liquid and powder diets

In my opinion, this type of diet is one of the worst offenders on the market. You replace all your food with sachets of powdered nutrients that you mix into a shake and take 3 times per day for 6 weeks, initially. Then, you reintroduce food for 1 meal and then up to 3 meals over a number of weeks (how many weeks depends totally on each individual), but almost always results in rapid weight gain.

You will have rapid weight loss at the very start – very rapid. Side effects may include fatigue, anaemia, bad skin, menstrual abnormality and a weakening of nails and hair, to such an extreme that hair has been known to fall out in clumps. Again, normally, you will regain the weight and more even more quickly than you lost it, as you aren't making any long-term changes.

Liquid diets offer little fibre and lack the important antioxidants found in fruits and vegetables. Does this sound healthy to you? Yet I am sure you know of someone who has tried it or maybe you have tried it yourself. There are several different versions of this diet on the market, all work off a very similar premise, no food and all shakes. If you take one important note from this whole book, this is it: These diets will damage your health.

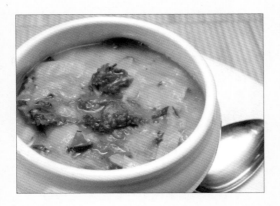

Cabbage soup

This is an age-old diet that has been around for a long, long time. It is a 7-to-14 day quick fix that is based around a fat-burning soup that helps to raise your metabolism as well as being very low in calories. There are several different versions of this diet and while you will lose weight quickly in the short term, after the week, you will put more weight back on when you return to eating food!

The most recent version of this diet that I have seen is used by doctors who want to perform surgery on patients that are too overweight. They will use this diet as a rapid weight loss solution, so that they can perform the surgery on the patients.

Juicing

Since Jason Vale made juicing popular a few years ago, it has gained a lot of fans. The benefits of juicing have been promoted for years and years and I must say that, in moderation or as part of a healthy diet, juicing can be very good for you. It is a great way to get nutrients into your body in their purest form. While it isn't sensible to replace food with juicing, there are certainly benefits to include it as part of your overall diet.

Do not to replace any meal with a juice, simply add a freshly squeezed juice that you have prepared yourself to a healthy meal, such as breakfast. Juices that you buy on the supermarket shelves have long shelf lives and very little nutritional value as they tend to be very high in sugar, with questionable health benefits. Most of the nutrients have been pasteurised out of the juice, which is what gives it the long shelf life.

KARL'S FRIGHTENING FACT

Some quick-fix diets reduce your calorific intake to under 600 calories! An average body needs around 2,000 calories a day to function normally.

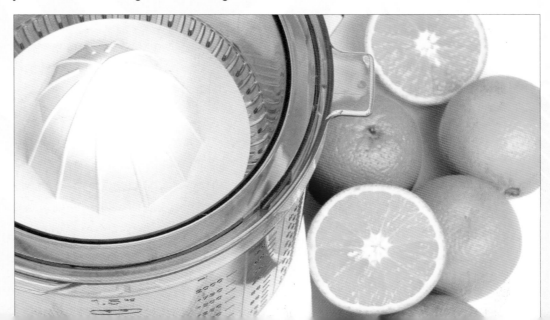

Now you understand how these different diets work, you have an educated opinion about them. No longer will these diets, or the different variations of the diets, that appear every January as quick-fix solutions confuse you.

In this book, you will learn how to eat real food, healthy food with no portion control, no limiting your food or no calorie counting. You will learn the reasons that your weight stabilises, which body type you have, which classes are good for you and which are doing you harm. You will finish this book with an educated opinion, ready to tackle your own goals. I am going to show you that real weight loss is achieved through eating healthy food and getting out there and doing some exercise.

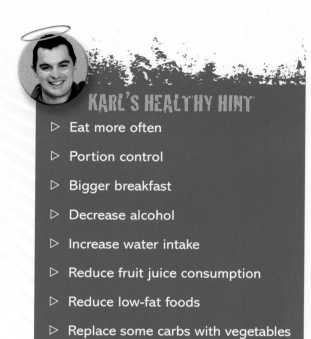

KARL'S HEALTHY HINT

▷ Eat more often

▷ Portion control

▷ Bigger breakfast

▷ Decrease alcohol

▷ Increase water intake

▷ Reduce fruit juice consumption

▷ Reduce low-fat foods

▷ Replace some carbs with vegetables

Glycemic index

Now that you know all about how not to eat, I am going to tell you about something you can use to help you eat for health, for life and for weight loss – the low glycemic index.

Here is the good news, to get real results that last for ever, you do not need to count calories, nor do you need to cut out any essential nutrient from your diet – and you don't need to eliminate that junk food that tastes so nice from your diet either. From my experience in the fitness industry, I have seen nearly every quick-fix diet going, and I have seen that they don't work. But I have also seen what does work and how to keep weight off. The way to do this is to simply follow the low gylcemic index way of eating. I know it sounds scary, but let's look at exactly what it is.

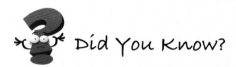
Did You Know?

Karl's simple explanation:

The glycemic index is a classification of the rise in sugar in your blood after you eat a certain type of food.

You may have heard of the glycemic index (GI) before, but may not have been able to understand exactly what it is about. It is simple and easy to do, so let's take a look.

Obviously, some foods cause a larger rise than others. Foods that cause your blood sugars to rise rapidly will lead to an increase in your weight as your body only uses around 30 per cent of the energy in that source, and stores the rest. Foods with a low glycemic index will keep your blood sugar level low and so your body uses more of the energy and less is stored in the body.

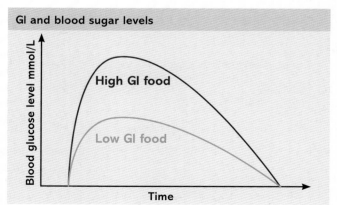

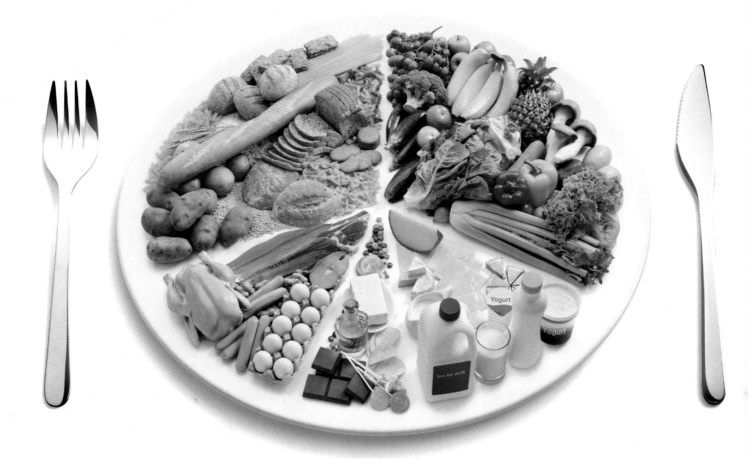

The typical Irish diet consists of foods that are higher up the glycemix index – which is one of the reasons why nearly half of Irish adults are overweight. Ever wonder why you get so hungry about 2 hours after your sugar-fuelled cereal in the morning? Or why you feel so good after that fizzy drink only to be absolutely knackered 2 hours later? This is all down to the fact that you're eating a high GI food.

Summary of glycemic index in foods

Type of food	Effect on blood sugar	Effect on weight	Effect on energy	Example	Effect on hunger
High glycemic index	Rapid increase	Increase	Rapid increase followed by a rapid decrease	Sugary, supposedly healthy cereal	Hungry 2 hours later
Low glycemic index	Slow increase	Steady decrease	Steady increase	Porridge	Feel full longer

The chart above shows you just how these foods work and the effect that they have on weight gain. If you feel knackered all day, have bad skin, have no zest for life at all and are constantly hungry, then take a look at the table above, it should be pretty easy to figure out why you feel the way you do.

Real Results

Glycemic food list

Below you will see the GI of many of your favourite foods. Ideally, the foods you eat should be below 50 – have a look through and see where foods that are in your diet rate!

Glycemic index list

Food	per 100g	Food	per 100g	Food	per 100g
Beer	110	Jam	65	Peas-dried (when cooked)	35
Potato (baked)	95	Melon	65	Raw carrots	35
Potato (chips)	95	Banana	65	Full-milk yoghurt	35
Puffed rice	95	Processed orange juice	65	Skimmed-milk yoghurt	35
Mashed potato	90	Raisins	65	Orange	35
Rice (pre-cooked)	90	White rice	60	Pear	35
Honey	90	Shortbread biscuits	55	Fig	35
Carrots cooked	85	Petit buerre biscuits	55	Apricots	35
Corn flakes	85	White pasta	55	Semi-skimmed milk	35
Popcorn	85	Unrefined flour	50	All Bran	30
Flour (white bread)	85	Buckwheat	50	Peaches	30
Rice cakes	85	Pancakes	50	Apples	30
Potato crisps	80	Sweet potato	50	Beans (haricot)	30
Baked beans (cooked)	80	Kiwi fruit	50	Beans (French)	30
Tapioca	80	Basmati rice	50	Brown lentils	30
Crackers	80	Brown rice	50	Cooked chickpeas	30
Pumpkin	75	Sorbet	50	Fruit preserve (without sugar)	30
Flour (baguettes)	75	Flour (pasta)	45	Dark chocolate	30
Watermelon	75	Bran (bread)	45	Green lentils	30
Flour (country-style bread)	70	Spaghetti	45	Split peas	22
Cereals (sugared)	70	Black bread	40	Cherries	22
Chocolate bars	70	Peas	40	Plums	22
Potato (peeled and boiled)	70	Grapes	40	Grapefruit	22
Sugar	70	Fresh orange juice	40	Fructose	22
Turnip	70	Fresh apple juice	40	Cooked soya	20
Cornflour	70	Rye bread	40	Peanuts	20
Maize	70	Unrefined flour (pasta)	40	Apricots (fresh)	20
Pre-cooked, non-stick rice	70	Kidney beans	40	Walnuts	20
Cola drinks	70	Unrefined flour (bread)	40	Onions	20
Noodles	70	Ice cream	40	Garlic	15
Brown flour (brown bread)	65	Chinese vermicelli	35	Green veg, lettuce, mushrooms	10
Potatoes (boiled in skin)	65	Corn on the cob	35	Tomatoes, aubergines, red peppers	10
Semolina	65	Quinoa (cooked)	35	Cabbage, broccoli	10

What foods should you be eating?

Are you ready to change how you feel? Get rid of that tiredness that plagues your day?

Now that you understand what glycemic index is about and what affects foods have on your body, let's introduce you to the food plans.

Breakfast

Breakfast is the most important meal of the day. Have you ever heard of the phrase: 'Breakfast like a king, lunch like a queen and dinner like a pauper'? This is an age-old saying that emphasises just how important breakfast is. Breakfast should be one of your biggest meals of the day, with lots of low GI carbohydrates to give you your fuel for the day ahead. You will be speeding up your metabolism, burning more calories naturally during the day, helping you to lose more weight. Your day will be more productive, more energetic and more fun as you will be brimming with energy! Simply put, cutting out breakfast is like driving a car without any fuel in it, you need to get the fuel in, so eat up! As you can see in the lists on page 59, aim to have nutritious cereals rather than most that you will find on the supermarket shelves.

Those cereals in the big boxes on the supermarket shelves are normally:

- ▶ High in sugar.
- ▶ High in salt.
- ▶ Low in nutritional value.
- ▶ Of little or no use to you.

So choose something healthy as a cereal and combine it with some brown bread toast which is full of healthy carbs.

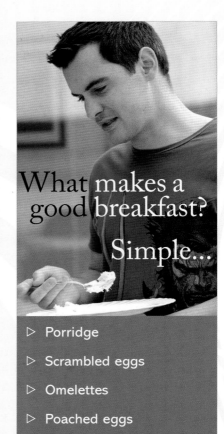

What makes a good breakfast? Simple...

- ▷ Porridge
- ▷ Scrambled eggs
- ▷ Omelettes
- ▷ Poached eggs
- ▷ Wholegrain or brown bread toast
- ▷ Low sugar granola or muesli/bran-based cereal

KARL'S FRIGHTENING FACT

Many orange juice products that we all see on supermarket shelves are often just full of sugar, they are concentrated to give the product a long shelf life, drastically reducing the nutritional value. Ask yourself this: how long would a litre of freshly squeezed orange juice last you if you squeezed it yourself at home?

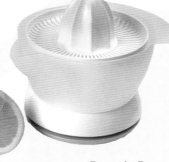

Real Results

Below you will see a table with three simple columns:

▸ **Recommended** These are the staples and main part of your diet, a total low GI food that will leave you feeling full and with plenty of energy. When you look at the list, you will see that they are foods you see every day, there's nothing scary here.

▸ **OK** Try to have these foods sometimes, they tend to be higher in sugar and will give you a higher blood-sugar level than the recommended foods.

▸ **Rarely** Try to avoid these foods, they are high in sugar and low in nutritional quality, best avoided except for that all-important treat day.

Does it look too easy to you? Trust me, it is simple to follow.

	Recommended		OK	Rarely
Fruit	Apple Pears Oranges Lemons Grapefruits Kiwis Peaches	Grapes Nectarine Cherries Prunes Strawberries Raspberries	Pineapples Papayas Mangos	Bananas Chestnuts
Bread Buns Cereals Sweet foods	Wholemeal bread Granary bread Wholegrain Ryvita Wholegrain bagels		Bagel with organic flour	Other bread or buns, other sweet sugar foods
Cereals Yeasts	Unrefined cereals without sugar Oat bran Wheatgerm Porridge Bran flakes/All Bran		Muesli without sugar Oat flakes Wheat bran	Sugary cereals Corn flakes Puffed rice Special K
Jams	Jams and marmalade without sugar or grape juice		Jam made with sucrose Hazelnut spread without sugar	Other jams, sweet spreads
Milk products	0% fat yoghurt Natural yoghurt Cottage cheese Soft white cheese Eggs Rice Dream/soya milk		Low-fat milk	Full-fat milk

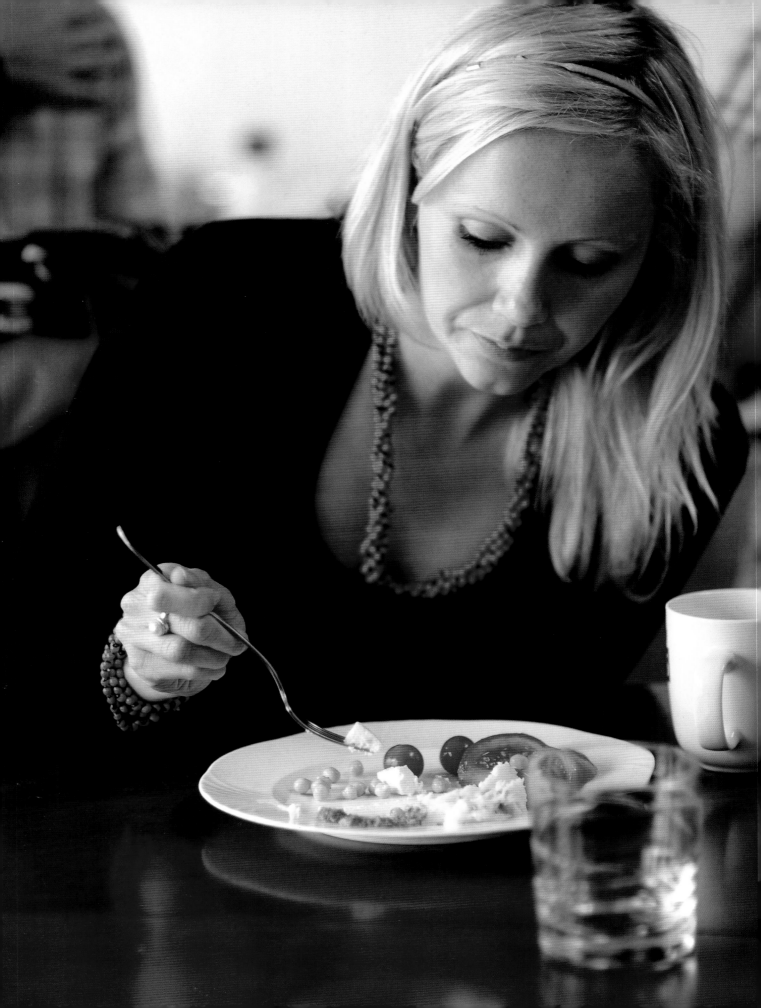

Lunches

Look good to you so far? The next list is for lunches, again we are keeping it simple, lots of yummy nutritious foods to eat, which are all low GI and healthy for you.

Bread

Choose from any of the following:

- Wholemeal pitta bread
- Wholemeal wraps
- Wholegrain bagels
- Soda bread
- Soya and linseed
- Wholegrain baguettes
- Brown bread with sunflower seeds, poppy seeds or multi-seeded

Karl's bread quality checker

Get your pan of bread, try to push both ends together. If you can push it very tight then you should put it back on the shelf. The higher the nutrient quantity, the harder it will be to push together.

Fillings

Any combination of the following:

- Sundried tomatoes, mozzarella and green salad leaves.
- Chopped chicken, sweetcorn, onion and fromage frais.
- Sliced egg, lettuce, red pepper and tomato.
- Feta cheese, rocket, tomato and red onion.
- Ham or chicken salad.
- Hummus, lettuce, peppers and onion.
- Cottage cheese.
- Turkey and cranberry sauce.
- Tuna, lettuce, red onion, peppers and sweetcorn.
- Smoked salmon with fresh lemon and cracked pepper.
- Baked beans (on toast, rather than as a sandwich).

Remember! no creamy dressings or mayonnaises with the above.

KARL'S FRIGHTENING FACT

White bread has virtually no nutritional value. It is air and starch. See what happens when you push both ends of a white sliced pan together. Companies are even dyeing the white bread brown now as it is cheaper to do!

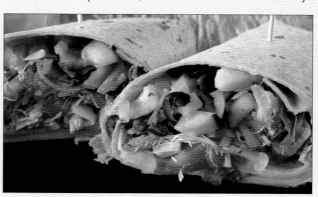

Soup and soda bread

Soup is fantastic for you and is full of nutrients but ensure that no cream has been added! Try to make your own as you know exactly what's gone into making it!

Snacks

Here is a suggestion about what to eat as snacks in between meals. You should be having a mid-morning snack and a mid-afternoon snack designed to provide balanced amounts of carbohydrates, protein and healthy fat for a low-moderate GI diet.

▸ Wholemeal scone with a little butter and jam.

▸ Low-fat yoghurt.

▸ Handful of nuts.

▸ Pumpkin/sunflower seeds.

▸ Wholegrain Ryvita.

▸ Fresh fruit.

▸ Smoothies, if they are home made.

▸ Dried fruit, nuts and raisins.

KARL'S FRIGHTENING FACT

Generally, the longer a shelf life a food has, the lower its nutritional value. Food is made to be eaten, not to last for weeks on end. To make food last, preservatives and additives need to be added, often replacing the nutrients. Try to eat fresh wholesome food for health!

Have you planned your breakfast yet? Picked out a nutritious lunch for yourself, all this talk of food might just be making you hungry!

Once a week aim to have a treat day!

This is your splurge day, have that pizza that you love so much, or the fish and chips from the local takeaway that always tastes so nice. This is why my plan is for real-life living. You are never going to cut out junk food from your diet for life, simply because it tastes so good. By having a treat day once a week, you are allowing yourself to have this food and you are also helping to speed up your metabolic rate. By eating food that your body isn't used to, your metabolism has to speed up to break it down. In the longer term, this will lead to a faster metabolism, meaning that you will burn more calories during the day.

Karl has been our personal trainer since 2006 – we believe we are the first husband and wife team that Karl has supervised.

We have been married for twenty-six years and have four children, ranging in ages from fourteen to twenty-five. When we were both in our late forties, we stated exercising with Karl as we were conscious that we could no longer take our weight, fitness and general health for granted. Now we train together in the privacy of our own home in Castleknock, Dublin.

From 2006 to 2009, as we built up our general levels of fitness, we had two sessions with Karl every week, with each session lasting an hour. The sessions always started at 6.15 in the morning, which minimised the disruption to our already full days. In 2010, we reduced the number of sessions to a single workout every week as our objectives for the workout changed.

Initially, we both had similar goals, we wanted to achieve our recommended weight (as determined by our respective heights), to achieve our recommended sizes in inches for arms, chest, stomach, waist, thighs and lower legs (as determined by Karl), to tone and, most importantly, to increase our levels of fitness and well being as we approached our fifties.

Karl developed a number of exercise routines which complemented us both. The exercises were designed around our mutual objectives and organised in set patterns which allowed us complete them simultaneously. The exercises were concentrated on the thighs and legs (lower body), stomach and/or upper body and arms. Not having been in a gym for over twenty years we both found the exercises extremely tough and sometimes painful. Depending on the routine and which muscle groups were being exercised the recovery period varied from one to three days. As you would expect our individual capacity to perform such a variety of exercises differed widely in the beginning, each of us having different levels of fitness, strength and flexibility. However, under Karl's watchful eyes – and our mutual desire to support one another in the exercises we individually found tough – we both gradually mastered the routines. However, four years after we first started, we accept that Karl always has a new approach and/or exercise that is beyond us to begin with. However, this is the added challenge that keeps the routines both interesting and demanding.

Today, our objectives are based on maintaining the results we have achieved over the past four years. We have reached our recommended weight levels but still weigh in every month to maintain our focus on weight control. We are acutely aware that the ageing process has slowed our metabolism and all our hard work could be undone in a short period.

We are also pleased with our general fitness and stamina levels, both physically and mentally, particularly when contrasted with those of a similar age. Basically, we are in good shape and intend to stay that way.

Dinner

Below is the list for dinners. As always it's incredibly simple, nearly every type of food is there – all healthy. Browse the list and see if the normal components of your diet are included.

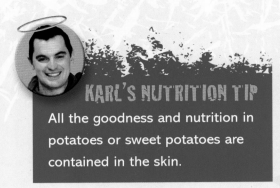

KARL'S NUTRITION TIP
All the goodness and nutrition in potatoes or sweet potatoes are contained in the skin.

Vegetables	Fish	Meat	Fowl	Other
Asparagus	Smoked salmon	Beef	Chicken	Goat's cheese
Tomatoes	Sole	Veal	Turkey	Cottage cheese
Cucumber	Sardines	Pork	Goose	Eggs
Artichokes	Mackerel	Mutton	Duck	Quorn
Peppers	Herring	Lamb	Pheasant	Brown pasta
Celery	Anchovies	Ham	Avoid skin	Brown rice
Mushrooms	Tuna	Avoid fatty cuts of meat as lean meat is far healthier		Sweet potato
French beans	Prawns			Tofu
Leeks	Scallops			
Cabbage	Lobster			
Cauliflower	Caviar			
Gherkins	Crab			
Avocado	Squid			
Bean sprouts	Oysters			
Lettuce	Avoid breaded or battered fish			
Watercress				
Broccoli				
Lentils				
Chick peas				

If your normal diet consists of the above foods, and you're wondering why you have put on weight, more than likely it will be down to the sauces that you are serving with your food. These can contain an amazing amount of fat and sugar and I will teach you how to read labels later in this section. Try to avoid sauces that are cream based; these are the real killers when it comes to a healthy diet. When eating salads, avoid the creamy mayonnaise-based dressings and simply switch to oil-based dressings, such as balsamic vinegar and olive oil.

Putting on weight

Many of my clients have the unenviable task of struggling to put on weight. They have difficulty with this despite trying everything and eating everything – and it can be a soul-destroying problem. It is normally due to a very fast metabolism that just burns up every calorie that is eaten. I know it sounds like a great problem to have but, believe me, it is equally as hard as being overweight. If you know someone who wants to put on weight, get them to try my method.

Basically to put on weight you need to dramatically increase your food intake. Because of the fact that your metabolism is so high, you need to be eating every 2 to 3 hours. Each meal should contain at least one, but ideally two, portions of protein. It is not just the amount of food that is important but they type of food that you eat. You want to be building muscle mass and in order to do that, you need protein. If you struggle to find time, try some protein shakes which provide an easy convenient way to get your protein in. There is a big debate about which is the best type of protein powder to get whey or casein. From my experience, I have to recommend whey protein.

In combination with eating protein every 2 to 3 hours, you need to be doing resistance exercises. The big difference with people who want to lose weight and those who want to put on weight is in the gym. To put on weight, you need to drop your reps from 5 to 10 and increase the sets to between 3 to 5. Try to pick 2 exercises per body part and the focus is on lifting heavier weights with a slightly bigger break in between sets.

Combining these two methods will lead to weight gain in even those with the highest metabolism. It's simple and it works, what more could you want? Ideally, you should be aiming to gain close to a pound of weight per week, slow and steady is the way forward in terms of keeping the weight on on a long-term basis.

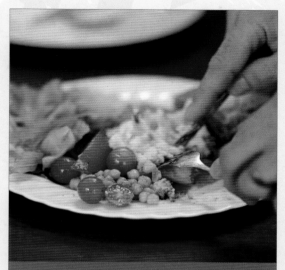

Karl's guide to eating out healthily

But what about eating out in restaurants?' I hear you ask. I love my food too, and I really love eating out in restaurants! The good news is that you can eat out and still lose weight! You simply need to be sensible. Aim to keep your starters simple – and salad or soup based. If you are steering away from these, then make it protein-based without the breadcrumbs or deep-fried coating! For your main meal aim to have plenty of protein-based foods, with the sauces on the side, stick to oil as opposed to creamy dressings and go for the salad as opposed to the potatoes or chips. Skip the dessert and you are home and dry!

If you are going to be healthy for life then you should be able to eat out, enjoy your food and enjoy life, just be sensible about it!

How much should you eat?

Many diets discuss portion control and limiting how much you actually eat. While this can be important, many people get confused about how much of each nutrient that they are allowed. I tend to recommend that as long as you are eating healthy foods, you can, within reason, eat until you feel full. It would be different if you were eating fish and chips every night, but if it is healthy then having a little bit extra won't do you any harm at all. For example 250 grams of white pasta isn't good for you, while 250 grams of brown pasta is full of fibre and totally healthy. It is important to remember that the food that you buy is not necessarily a portion, it will more often than not contain several portions of food, so remember to keep an eye on the label and to eat actual portions not the whole packet.

There you have the food plan, it really is that simple. Making the switch to low glycemic index foods is the healthy way to lose weight.

Common food errors

Eating too fast

Maybe it's something to do with the famines that we've had, but Irish people are terrible for devouring meals that are put in front of them. Eating too quickly puts the body under a lot of strain, so much so that it can't digest the food you've just eaten. You get what I call the Christmas effect, where you body shuts down in order to digest the food. Ever wonder why you fall asleep after a huge meal? That is your body shutting down, you have eaten so much so quickly that your body puts you to sleep so it can work to break down the food. To avoid this, put your knife and fork down between each mouthful, taste your food and let your body digest it.

Drinking too much with meals

Another Irish trait here. By drinking too much with your meals, you're diluting the enzymes in your stomach that help to digest your food and break it down. Some people recommend not drinking for an hour before and after you meal, I think that it is slightly extreme! I would advise not drinking too much with your meal, try to make that one glass last your entire meal.

Not chewing your food

We are born with teeth which are there to break down food but 60 per cent of the time, we don't use them enough! By chewing your food more, you make life a whole lot easier for your body. Food is broken down so it's easier to digest and extract nutrients from. Aim to chew your food for at least 10 seconds with each mouthful, ideally a little more if possible!

Food labels

Food labels are a legal requirement put in place by the government to tell you exactly how much energy is in the food you are eating, where the energy comes from and all of the ingredients that are in the food.

While it is great to have all this information, most people aren't sure how to read and decipher a food label – it can look so confusing that people just don't look at them. If you can learn to read food labels, then you will know straight away how healthy or unhealthy a product is.

Here is the big question: what is the most important piece of information on a food label?

Take a look at this label. Which nutrient is the most important? Many people think that it is energy, telling you how many calories are in the food. Fat is often another popular choice, people link the fat content of a label with fat on their bodies. Not so. The most important one in my opinion is the sugars value. Products that have versions that are low in fat or fat free tend to have a much higher sugar value that the normal version of that product.

Typical Values	Per 100g	Per ½ can	GDA*
Energy - kJ	230kJ	461kJ	
- kcal (Calories)	54kcal	109kcal	1800
Protein	1.8g	3.5g	24g
Carbohydrate	11.3g	22.6g	220g
(of which sugars)	(4.2g)	(8.4g)	85g
Fat	0.2g	0.4g	70g
(of which saturates)	(Trace)	(Trace)	20g
Fibre	0.5g	1.1g	15g
Sodium	0.1g	0.3g	1.4g
Salt equivalent	0.4g	0.7g	4g

*Guideline Daily Amounts for 5-10 year old children.

WHY IS SUGAR SO BAD?

▷ It is a highly processed food with no nutritional value.

▷ It is bad for teeth/oral health.

▷ It will force your body to release insulin which promotes the storage of fat.

▷ Sugar gives your body a quick fix in terms of energy, followed by a big energy low.

▷ While sugar is contained in fruit, it is a different form of sugar, being natural as opposed to processed.

▷ Diets high in sugar can lead to bad skin and spots.

▷ Sugar can lead to hyperactivity and depression.

▷ It's addictive.

Sugar is in most things we eat, even in foods that we think are healthy. Many probiotic drinks taste so good because they are high in sugar, containing as many as 3 spoonfuls of sugar per small bottle. Fizzy drinks contain as many as 10 spoonfuls!

I am not suggesting that you eliminate sugar from your diet totally, as that would be virtually impossible. Aim to get your sugar from as natural a source as possible, such as fruit or honey. Or when you are reading a label, aim to have sugar values less than 40 per cent of the carbohydrate value. I know it sounds complicated, but take a look at the following.

Product	Carbohydrate	Sugar	Good/Bad
1	100	75	Bad
2	100	35	Good

It really is this simple, when you are reading a food label, look out for this element alone and you will be healthier as a result.

Food planning

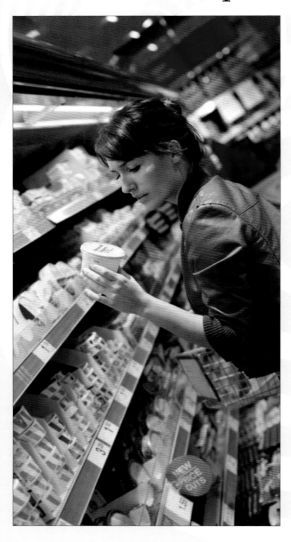

One element that is so often overlooked when trying to lose weight is planning. A great lecturer I once had always said that, 'Failing to plan is planning to fail', and this couldn't be more true.

You should always aim to get one big food shop done per week, stocking your kitchen full of all the foods that are low GI. By doing this, you are making life so much easier for yourself. If the healthy foods are there, then you will eat them, if not then your will be so much more tempted to eat junk or to order that high-calorie takeaway. Try put one day aside to get the food shopping done and life will become so much easier!

Here are some other things to take into consideration when eating:

▸ Eat up to 5 meals per day, with smaller portions.

▸ Eat until you feel satisfied.

▸ Vary your food as this helps to keep you interested.

▸ Avoid sugary drinks.

▸ Relax at meal times, try and enjoy your food.

▸ Chew your food.

By eating regular meals, you won't feel the need to snack a lot during the day. You will have increased energy levels, as these foods won't give you a huge increase followed by a decrease in your blood sugar.

Cooking methods

Throw away that deep-fat fryer if it still exists in your home. How you cook your food is equally as important as the type of food that you are eating. There is no point thinking that you are being healthy by buying fish if you are putting it into the deep-fat fryer with a thick layer of batter on it! A product of a bygone era, deep-fat frying is one of the worst methods of cooking your food. Below are three healthier ways to cook.

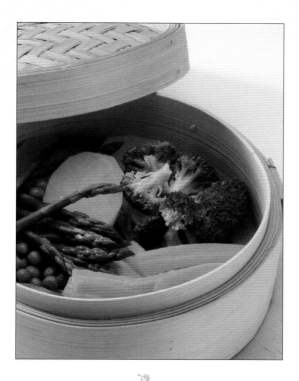

Karl's planning tip

Get out that pen and paper and write it down. A food diary will help you to keep track of your food intake and increase your chances of succeeding!

Steaming

Steaming is basically cooking food in an enclosed environment using steam. It seals in the flavour of the food as well as all the nutrients. It is especially good for fish as it doesn't dry out the fish and you don't need to add any fats to it to cook in. Steamers are available nationwide and are extremely cheap. If you want tasty, healthy food, then this is one of the easiest ways to get it.

Many people think that it takes too long to cook this way, but steaming fish can take between 8 to 15 minutes to steam, meat can take longer and vegetables generally take close to 10 minutes.

Stir frying

This is just cooking food at a very high heat for a short space of time. The food should be cut into small pieces and you can stir fry using a wok or a pan. Woks are great as the sloping sides make it easier for the food to cook as it won't spill over the side as you churn it. But take note, you need to stir the food continuously to ensure that everything gets cooked well. Literally everything and anything can be cooked in a stir fry, it's healthy and easy to do, less than 10 minutes will give you a great, healthy, nutritious meal.

George Foreman grilling

The modern answer for a world that cooks less and less. We have George Foreman to thank for the success of grills in the past 10 years, as soon as he put his name to the product (something that Hulk Hogan turned down), they literally sold millions across the globe! The beauty of the grill is that it cooks pretty much anything, using no fat-based oils and it drains all of the fat from a product too. Leaving you with a quick healthy meal. Most foods cook in under 10 minutes and literally anyone can use one.

Microwaving

After talking about healthy ways to cook, now let's look at a method that, in my opinion, you shouldn't use.

I am a firm believer that microwaves damage your health and shouldn't be used at all. So what if they lower the cooking time of your favourite dish? Are you willing to eat something that, when you take it out of the oven, will continue cooking for an average of 30 minutes – even as you eat it! That delicious microwaved meal that tastes so good while you are eating it is still cooking all the way into your stomach – the same thing happens with food that is reheated too. This is just one of the side effects of microwave cooking amongst the vast research that has been done over the past 40 years.

Like anything, there are two opinions to microwaving, mine is based on how I feel after I eat microwaved food, which I hasten to add is only when a restaurant serves me a microwaved dish! I do ask the waiters of any restaurant I eat in if their food is microwaved and if they tell me it is, I don't eat there!

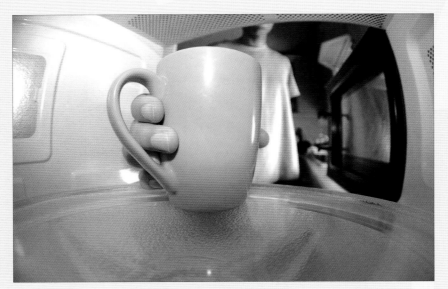

My personal experience isn't the only thing upon which my opinion is based. I have seen how the health of clients, who were suffering various conditions because they were eating a diet laden with microwaved food, has improved when they have thrown their microwaves away. I am not a scientist or a physicist, my opinions are simply based on real life, real stories and real people.

Microwave research findings

Below are further findings from research conducted as early as 1957 in Russia (the Russian government banned microwaves until 1976) to a 1989 study undertaken in Switzerland by Dr Hans Ulrich Hertel.. The points below are taken from *www.healthychoices.co.uk*, when they found the following:

▷ Continually eating food processed from a microwave oven causes long term – permanent – brain damage by 'shorting out' electrical impulses in the brain (de-polarising or de-magnetising the brain tissue).

▷ The human body cannot metabolise (break down) the unknown by-products created in microwaved food.

▷ Male and female hormone production is shut down and/or altered by eating microwaved foods continually.

▷ The effects of microwaved food by-products are residual (long term and permanent) within the human body.

▷ Minerals, vitamins and nutrients of all microwaved food is reduced or altered so that the human body gets little or no benefit from them, or the human body absorbs altered compounds that cannot be broken down.

▷ Some minerals in vegetables are altered into cancerous free-radicals when cooked in microwave ovens.

▷ Microwaved foods cause stomach and intestinal cancerous growths (tumours). This may explain the rapidly increased rate of colon cancer in America and Europe.

▷ The eating of microwaved foods over an extended period of time causes cancerous cells to increase in human blood.

▷ Continual ingestion of microwaved food causes immune system deficiencies through lymph gland and blood serum alterations.

▷ Eating microwaved food causes a loss of memory, concentration, emotional instability and decreases intelligence.

The fact that microwaving produces carcinogens is not new information and is something that is supported by research worldwide.

Like so many topics, there are those who will disagree with these conclusions. From my experience, I am a firm believer that microwaves are bad for your health. I am not suggesting that you, on the basis of this information, instantly change your mind, but I hope that it will make you think and do your own research to see what you feel about the whole area. If you eat a lot of microwaved food at the moment, how do you feel now? If you want to test any of the theories above, why not try not using your microwave for 2 weeks and see how you feel then? It can't hurt? I promise you that you will feel healthier, have improved skin and more energy – amongst a whole lot of other benefits for you and your body. Go on, try it for a few weeks and see what a difference it makes to your body.

Fluids

'But what about fluid?' I hear you ask. As with every area of diet, this is extremely confusing.

Below are the simple facts. Water in your diet does the following:

▸ Increases your energy levels.

▸ Decreases your hunger, you are often thirsty rather than hungry.

▸ Regulates your body temperature.

▸ Increases your concentration levels.

▸ Aids fat loss through increased toilet breaks.

Many people don't get enough water during the day and spend much of their time dehydrated. A simple dehydration test is the fact that you shouldn't be thirsty at all during the day, thirst is a sign that your body is very dehydrated, so get some fluid into you asap if you are!

The ingredients in a Burger King milkshake are:

Amyl acetate, amyl butrate, amyl valerate, anethol, anisyl formate, benzyl acetate, benzyl asobutyrate, butric acid, cinnamyl, isobutyrate, cinnamyl valerate, cognac essential oil, diacetyl, dipropyl,ketone,ethyl acetate, ethyl amyl ketone, ethyl butrate, ethyl cinnemate, ethyl heptoanate, ethyl heptylate, ethyl lactate, ethyl methylphenyl-glycidate, ethyl nitrate, ethyl propionate, ethyl valerate, heliotropin, hydroxyphenyl-2-butanone, alpha-ionone, isobutyl anthranilate, isobutyl, butyrate, lemon essential oil, maltol, 4-methylacetophenone, methyl anthranilate, methyl benzoate, methyl cinnamate, methyl heptine carbonate, methyl naphthyl ketone, methyl salicylate, mint essential oil, neroli essential oil, nerolin, neryl isobutyrate, orris butter, phenethyl alcohol, rose rum ether, y-undecalactone, vanillin and solvent.

(Eric Schlosser, 2003)

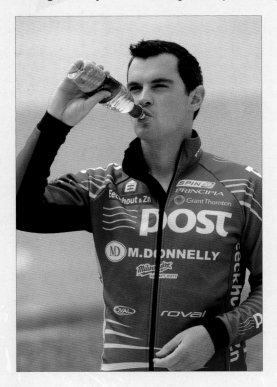

Water is essential for health and also in helping you to lose weight! Many times when you feel hungry, you are actually thirsty. Without sounding like a nun of the mill advisor, you should aim to drink 2 litres of water per day, depending on your activity levels. Obviously, if you are more active, the chances are that you will need to get more water into your day. The easiest way to do this is to get a 2-litre bottle and fill it at the start of the day. By the end of the day, the bottle should be empty! No glasses, no confusion, just a simple visual of having to have the bottle empty by the end of the day.

There was some bad press given to water over the past year or two, with people who drank too much actually dying. This was down to yet another quick-fix diet that told you to drink 6 or more litres per day, which caused a swelling in the brain. So stick to your 2 litres and you will be safely hydrated.

Real Results

Another point to note is that coffee and tea don't count towards your overall limit. The 2 litres need to come from pure, non-sparkling H_2O, coffee and tea contain caffeine and many herbal teas contain caffeine too, so stick to your water.

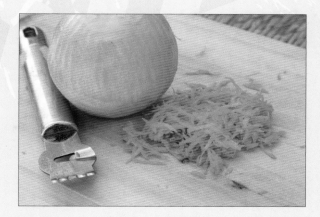

If you find it a little plain then feel free to add some fruit into the bottle, not the sugary syrup that you can buy in the shops, but actual fruit. This will add some flavour to the water and may make it easier for you to drink.

Alcohol

An essential part of any food section! Here is the good news, I won't be saying that you can never drink alcohol again. I will be simply showing you the effects of alcohol and what the best types to have are. Alcohol is basically a central nervous system depressant, although in smaller amounts it may appear to have a mild stimulant effect.

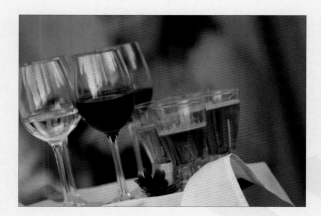

Different people react to alcohol differently, but the effects generally depend on a number of factors, including the type and quantity of alcohol you consume, your age, weight and gender and body chemistry, the food in your stomach and, of course, your drinking experience.

I am a terrible lightweight when it comes to drinking as I only drink a handful of times a year. I find that the post-night-out effects are so damaging to my body and mind that I prefer to limit them.

The side effects after drinking can be:

▸ Depression

▸ A non-stop hunger for junk food

▸ Fatigue

▸ Irritability

▸ Lack of motivation

And these are just *some* of the side effects.

Think about how you felt after your last big night out. The effects can last for up to 3 days. Now I am not saying that you shouldn't drink ever again, but try to introduce the very non-Irish notion of moderation! A glass of wine with dinner may actually be good for you, but obviously several won't be! In terms of health and weight loss, different types of alcohol have a big effect on your body. Let's take a look.

Drink	Nutrient	Effect	Karl's tip	Calories
Beer	Yeast	Bloating Beer belly	Has been found to contain minute traces of oestrogen	200-300 per pint
Wine	Sugar	Too much can lead to insulin production, increasing fat storage	Red tends to be the healthier of the 3 types	120-150 per glass
Champagne	Sugar	Can cause gaseousness	You tend to drink less because of the bubbles	65-80 per glass
Spirits	Varies		The mixers do the damage, as they are normally high in sugar	40-50 per measure
Cider	Sugar	Bloating	Varies, but organic is best	200–300 per pint

Take a minute to digest the information above!

The first startling fact is that beer contains minute traces of oestrogen. In women, this is not so much of an issue, in men, however, this is a totally different story. Have you ever wondered why men who drink a lot of beer develop man boobs? Literally soft tissue begins to droop in a breast-like form, getting bigger and bigger as the years go by. Well gentlemen, this is because your body is getting confused and begins to think it's a woman, because of the oestrogen being ingested from the beer, even in such minute forms.

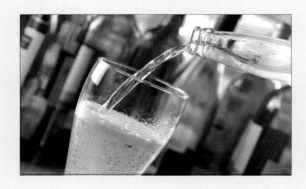

High beer consumption also leads to a beer belly, an area of bloated, yet very firm tissue around the stomach area, initially it will be quite soft and then as the years go by it gets harder and harder. This is caused by the yeast fermenting in the gut, the more beer you drink, the harder it is going to get. Even the lower calorie version of beer and cider contain high amounts of sugar and yeast, it may have fewer calories but it won't be much better for you.

Cider has similar effects, though this is more because of the very high sugar content rather than the yeast. As a cider drinker myself, I notice the effects any time that I do drink.

Wine although a much healthier option is still very high in sugar. Sugar causes your body to release insulin which promotes fat storage in the body.

It is very easy to tell what people drink, by looking at the type of fat they have around their midriff. Wine drinkers tend to develop what I call the wine wobble. Soft fatty tissue that will literally wobble when you move! As I said before, 1 glass with dinner won't cause this, but 1 bottle with dinner will! Red wine is certainly the healthier of the 3 types as it is full of antioxidants that are good for your body and the effects of anti-ageing. Moderation is the key!

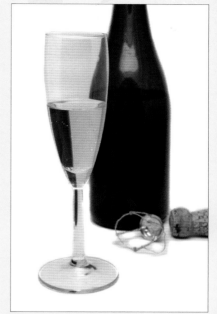

Champagne is always my recommended drink for anyone who is trying to lose weight and wants to have a few drinks at the weekend. It is so much lower in calories, with around 75 calories per glass. Because it is full of bubbles, you tend to drink less of it as it's hard to drink quickly. It also tends to be quite strong in alcoholic content, another reason that you will want to drink less.

Amongst my younger clients, especially those I meet during my lectures, spirits and mixers tend to be the drink of choice – I have met so many clients who would easily have ten shorts and mixers on a night out. This is a fascinating area, while the alcohol may be low in calorie terms, the mixers certainly aren't and are full of sugar, leading to the soft fatty skin around the waist area. Shorts, themselves, are very low in calories, but try to stick to tonic as the mixer of choice, the fizzy drink mixers will contain between 5 and 7 spoons of sugar per mixer, if you're having 10 drinks per night, then that's at least 50 spoonfuls of sugar on each night out!

Long-term heavy alcohol use can have the following effects on the body:

▸ Heart damage

▸ High blood pressure and stroke

▸ Liver damage

▸ Cancers of the digestive system

▸ Other digestive system disorders (e.g. stomach ulcers)

▸ Sexual impotence and reduced fertility

▸ Increased risk of breast cancer

▸ Sleeping difficulties

▸ Brain damage with mood and personality changes

▸ Concentration and memory problems

Alcohol is an intrinsic part of Irish culture. We will probably need to keep this in your diet if you are trying to be healthy and slim for life. By cutting it out, chances are that you will binge drink more. Moderation is the key as well as the type of alcohol that you choose to drink.

I can't make this choice for you, I can simply show you the real information for each type that's out there. Make it simple to understand and then the choice is up to you.

Men in particular are terrible at making fun of each other when they don't drink, it's seen as a very non-masculine trait, even more so if you choose not to have the pint of beer. Next time that happens, ask your friends if they too want man boobs, or the trouser-bursting, belt-breaking bloated stomach that they are going to get.

Drinking while pregnant

What about drinking while pregnant? This is not an area that I am personally qualified to make recommendations about, but on completing research for this book, it became apparent that there are some general guidelines that most experts seem agreed on. This is what the American Pregnancy Association has to say about drinking alcohol during pregnancy:

When you consume alcohol, so does your baby. Alcohol freely passes through the placenta to your baby. Drinking alcohol during pregnancy increases the chance that a baby will be born affected by a Fetal Alcohol Spectrum Disorder (FASD). Fetal Alcohol Spectrum Disorders (FASD) are the full spectrum of birth defects that are caused by pre-natal alcohol exposure. These effects are life-long and irreversible. The good thing is that they are 100 per cent preventable.

As with all the information in this book, it is for you to make up your own mind. My opinion based upon my own research is that is safer and healthier – for you and your baby – not to drink when you are pregnant.

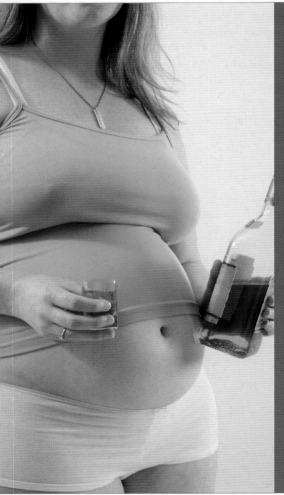

It is in a child's best interests for a prospective mother not to drink alcohol while pregnant due to the risk of developmental brain disorders to the child. Yet 2 out of 3 women in Ireland continue to drink alcohol during their pregnancies. The advice from the country's Chief Medical Officer is clear:

'Given the harmful drinking patterns in Ireland and the propensity to binge drink, there is a substantial risk of neurological damage to the foetus resulting in Foetal Alcohol Spectrum Disorders (FASD). Therefore, it is in the child's best interest for a pregnant woman not to drink alcohol during pregnancy. Drinking heavily during pregnancy can also increase the chances of complications during pregnancy and childbirth, as well as increasing the risk of miscarriage and stillbirth. A leaflet on women and alcohol published by the Health Promotion Unit advises that there is no known safe level of alcohol use during pregnancy and that women should stop drinking during this time. It makes the following points:

▷ More than 3 drinks a day increases the risk of miscarriage.

▷ More than 12 drinks in a week increases the risk of premature birth.

▷ Sudden high levels of alcohol damages the developing brain.'

Alcohol Ireland

Detoxing

By reducing the amount of sugar in your diet, you are going to have a sugar detox, this can manifest itself in many ways but the common symptoms are:

- Headaches
- Spots
- Rashes
- Nausea
- Low energy

These are all short-term conditions that come about as your body eliminates the waste and sugar. This is simply your body detoxing, real detoxing. And, I'm afraid, that real detoxing can have these effects on you – patches won't do the same thing.

Depending on the level of sugar that was in your diet, it can take 1 to 4 days to detox completely but, believe me, when it passes, you will feel better than ever. When you are through the detox blues, you will have:

- More energy
- Better skin
- Better concentration levels
- Better moods

Detoxing is a big buzz word in the fitness industry, even more so at New Year! But what is the idea behind it? Why do we do it? Detoxing is done to eliminate all the waste from our bodies and to try get our systems to return to their normal state.

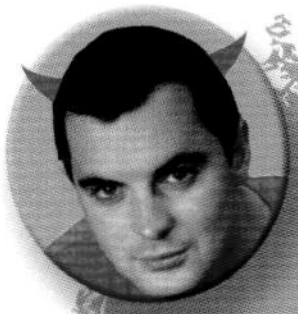

The processed foods that we eat are not good for our bodies, causing any number of problems, detoxing is done to try to flush these out. Sometimes people detox for weight loss, as you will also lose weight doing it. As always, companies have tried to capitalise on this, with quick-fix solutions sold that offer no discomfort, such as the foot detox patches. But this isn't the same, or as good, as real detoxing, which will have some side effects such as:

KARL'S FRIGHT'ENING FACT

Your digestive system runs 48 to 72 hours behind, so when eating your next meal just remember that it will be in your body for up to 3 days

- Headaches
- Spots
- Nauseousness
- Rashes
- Tiredness
- Irritability
- Lack of motivation
- Increased sweat rates

These symptoms may last between 3 to 7 days, depending on just how bad your diet was before you started the detox.

Without getting all Gillian McKeith on you, you might find that your stools are very dark — I have even come across cases where they were almost white. During the detox period, your body is eliminating all the waste that has built up, self-regulating itself. You will be less bloated, more radiant, healthier and will feel stronger than before.

There are a few methods that I have come across to detox.

The cabbage soup

Also used as a quick-fix diet solution, this has also been known to have detox qualities. It consists of eating a vegetable-based broth several times per day, different versions also use food combining.

Juicing

This is another very common method. You simply juice, yourself of course, oranges or other fruit. You drink every time that you are hungry — which can be up to 5 litres of juice per day. While the juice is acidic, it can be very effective as a detox tool. Another version of this is also done using fruit, eaten whole as opposed to juiced. Fruits such as pears are fantastic for this.

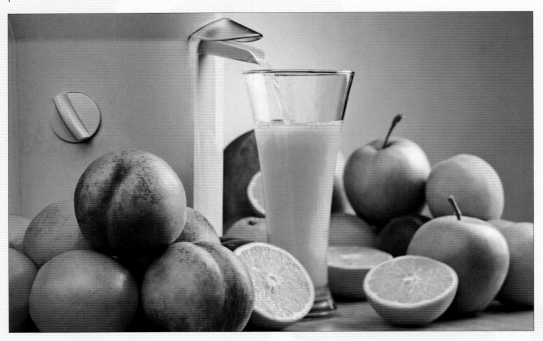

Colonic irrigation

This is also a form of detoxing. While it may be controversial, I must say that I am a fan of it. I have recommended it to many of my clients and seen great results. However, if you are getting it done, aim to have a clinical doctor perform the procedure rather than your beautician. I feel that doctors have more knowledge about the procedure and its effects.

Real Results

What is colonic irrigation? Put simply, water is passed through the rectum into the digestional tract which, when released, brings toxins and old faeces with it, this is repeated several times and, at the end, you will feel much better. It helps your body return to its normal digestive rhythm, reducing bloating and constipation. It is important to remember to drink plenty of water after having this done, and to include plenty of natural yoghurt with lactobacilus and other natural enzymes in it.

Cellulite: the curse of women and even men!

Cellulite basically refers to the dimpled appearance of the skin that some people have on their hips, thighs and buttocks, as well as, in more recent years, the back of their arms. This appearance is much more common in women than in men because of differences in the way fat, muscle and connective tissue are distributed in men and women's skin. The lumpiness of cellulite is caused by fat deposits that push and distort the connective tissues beneath skin. As the fat deposits increase in all the areas that cellulite appears, it has nowhere else to go so it pushes through the skin and creates that lumpiness.

Many people will tell you that cellulite has a genetic link or that there is nothing that you can do about it. Not in my opinion! The good news is that yes it can be improved! There are many expensive therapies, such as endimology, that can help reduce the effects of cellulite but I am going to show you best ways to reduce cellulite that are cheap and effective.

▷ **Processed foods:** Reduce the number of processed foods in your diet. Processed foods are high in fat and preservatives, two nutrients that, in my experience, have a direct link to cellulite.

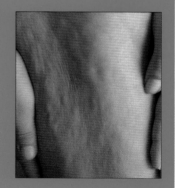

▷ **Water intake:** If you are trying to remove the toxins and fat from your body, then increasing your water intake will help, as you will be visiting the toilet more often, helping to excrete the toxins!

▷ **Exercise:** A mixture of cardiovascular and resistance exercise. This helps to tone the muscles in the area, leading to firmer muscles.

▷ **Ki Massage:** Massage helps to break down the fat cells that often become very hard as you get older. It can be sore, but when the fat has been broken down, the massage will automatically become softer, changing the texture of the cellulite.

Some say that there is no link between cellulite and diet. I have several clients that prove the opposite is true. One client in particular who prepares her own food and doesn't eat any processed foods at all. Who enjoys a glass of wine with dinner and some chocolate every now and again. This lady has the best arms and legs that you will ever see, toned, feminine and firm – she is the envy of women in their teens and twenties who would do anything for arms like hers. She has achieved her toned body by living a balanced life, doing some exercise and eating a healthy diet.

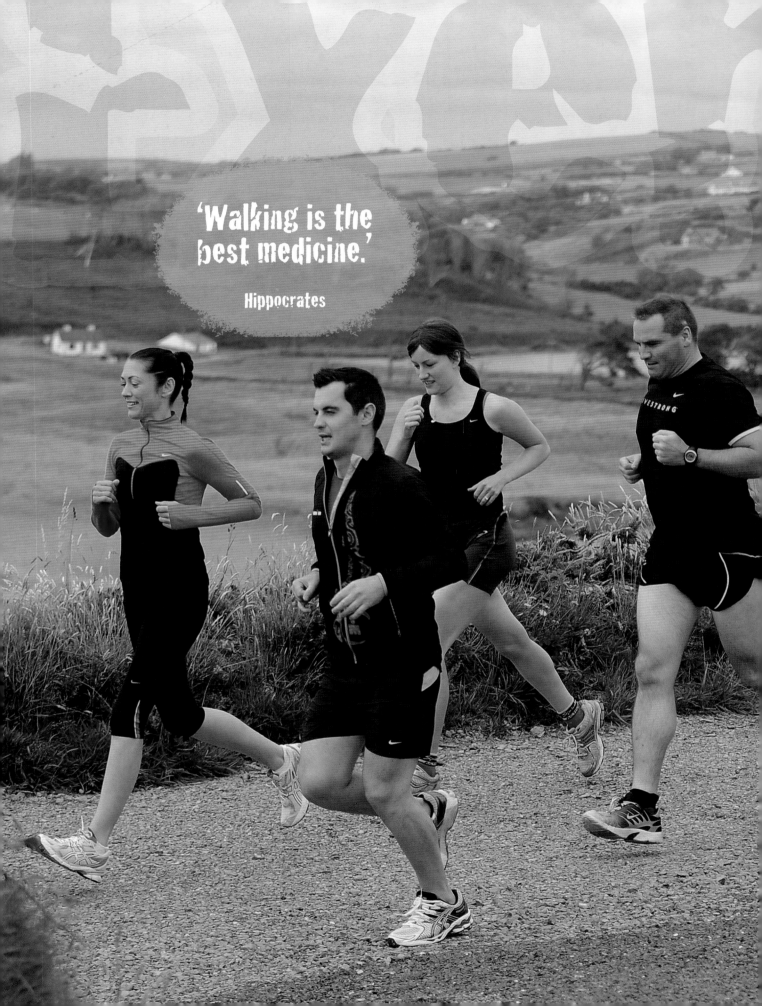

'Walking is the best medicine.'

Hippocrates

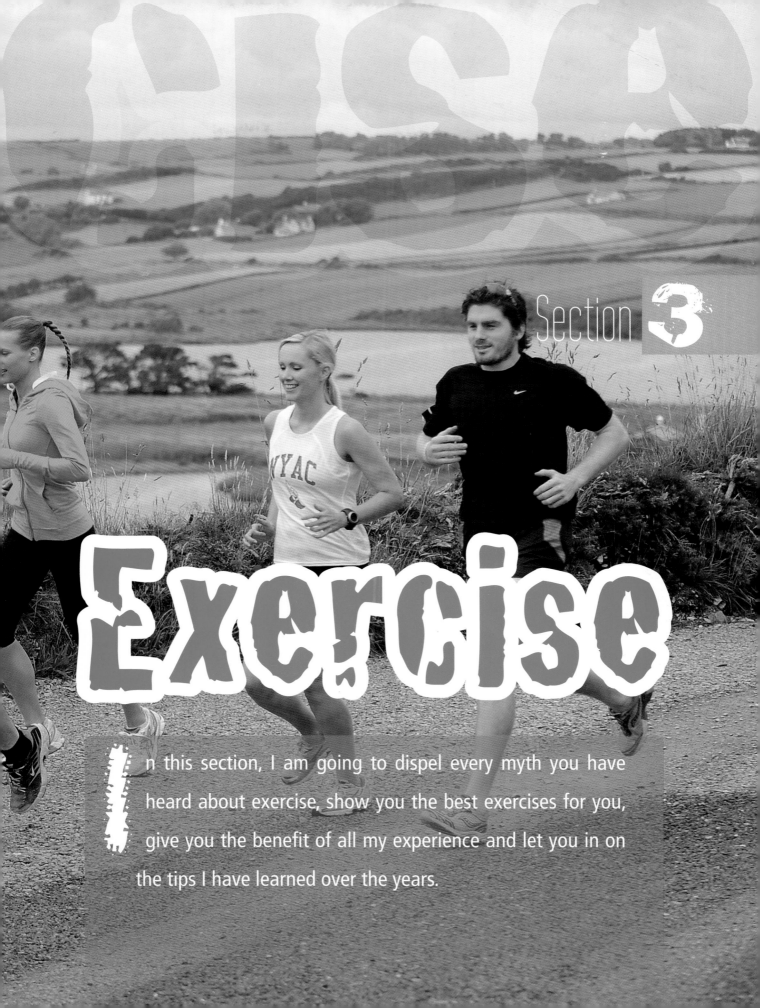

Exercise

In this section, I am going to dispel every myth you have heard about exercise, show you the best exercises for you, give you the benefit of all my experience and let you in on the tips I have learned over the years.

There are three components essential to real weight loss. The first is a **healthy diet**, the second is **cardiovascular exercise** and the third is **resistance training**. These three components will give you the healthiest, fittest, firmest body possible.

At first, exercise can often seem scary – like nearly every other area of the health industry – with lots of scary words and gyms full of people who look like they know what they are doing. I can promise you that it isn't frightening at all. Whether you are a beginner or have been training for several years, I am going to show you a workout that will give you beneficial results.

Want to train in your home? Great, there will be a workout for that. Need help with your running? I will show you how! Want to get amazing, longer-looking legs? Great, I love working on leg training with my clients and am going to share all – well maybe not all – but most of my leg-training secrets with you.

No matter what your fitness level is, you will find something in this section that will help you to take your training to the next level. As always, I am not into recommending fad exercises or certain things that I feel are totally useless. I will give you the facts and the real way to get the best results so that your results will last – this book is designed to get you fit for life not just for 6 weeks! Quick-fix exercise gimmicks will come and go, real exercises will last.

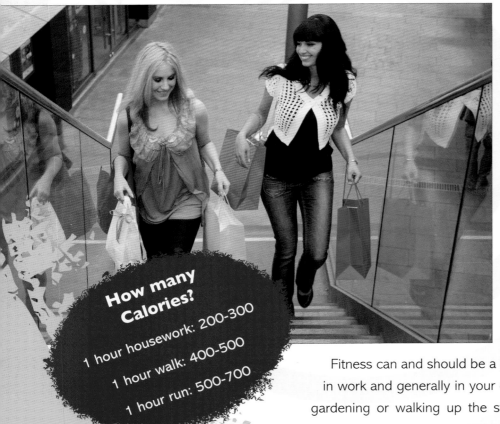

How many Calories?

1 hour housework: 200-300

1 hour walk: 400-500

1 hour run: 500-700

In this section, you will not find me relying on Swiss balls, Kettlebells or Power Plates, what you will find are exercises that anyone of any age can do to help them achieve results that will last. All you will need are 2 bottles of water and a mat. The reason that the 2 bottles of water work so well is that as you get stronger, you can just get heavier bottles. Easy! If you have 2 dumbbells at home, they will be perfect to use – if not, get those bottles of water and get yourself ready to go.

Fitness can and should be a part of your everyday life, at home, in work and generally in your day. Whether it's doing housework, gardening or walking up the stairs in a shopping centre, simply

Real Results

getting any exercise into your day will make a huge difference to your body and your mind. Don't be afraid to analyse your day, look at where you take the easy option and where you could change that to something that has more activity. Escalators and lifts are great examples of this, why not take the stairs instead and work your lungs, legs and upper body in the process? Every little bit helps in terms of movement and exercise, so try it tomorrow – today even – and feel the difference that it will make in your life.

Family fitness

I truly believe that the solution to this obesity epidemic lies with each and every family across Ireland. Yes, the government has much to do, as do the schools, but change must start at home and parents have a responsibility to teach their children habits that they will keep for the rest of their lives.

If you raise your child on McDonald's, chances are that's what they will continue to eat later in life. As ever, I am not suggesting a radical approach, simply limit those treats to once a week not every day, teach your children about food and the importance of it and get them moving. Children need to be exposed to the benefits of exercise, let those endorphins give them the feel-good factor early in life and chances are they will keep up the exercise for life! You have now made the decision that you want to change your family environment, great. Change can be hard to implement but stick with it. Now follow me.

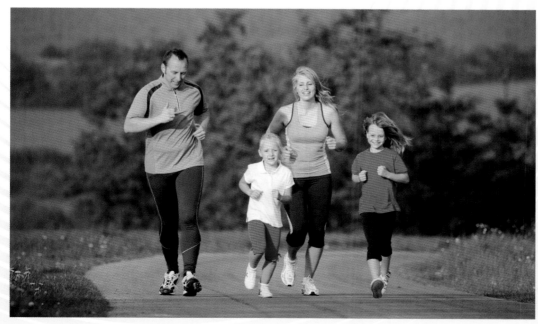

You need to set aside regular time for the family and stick to it. When this time is agreed, commit to using it for exercise or an outdoor activity. Why not take it in turns to choose what sport you do? This will ensure that everyone gets to do an exercise that they want to and it also makes it more fun. You may feel that everyone's schedule is too busy to fit in time to exercise, but even spending an hour over the course of a weekend is a good start. It can be easy to leave your children to be entertained by the television for a while whilst you get on with other things, but your children will love it if you take the time to do something active with them – so not only are they getting some exercise, but you will feel good too.

When playing sports as a family, I think that it is essential to emphasise the importance of playing for fun rather than playing to win. Children should not be pushed to their limit, it is about having fun and creating a feel-good factor.

In addition to setting aside the time to exercise, it is also important to analyse the kitchen in your home, if you stock it full of fruit and healthy food, then that's what will be eaten. Similarly, if you have Coke and chocolate, then that's what your family will eat! Treats are important in creating balance, but use them as that – a treat!

You may also have to learn the power of the word no! I think that a large part of the problem with childhood obesity is that parents are almost afraid of saying no to their children. If fizzy drinks are a problem in your house, then stop buying them and buy water instead! You are the parent and your role is to set the rules and lead by example. You are creating the habits and associations with food and exercise that your children will have for the rest of their lives, so why not aim to set good ones?

Now you know how to go about it, but what kind of exercise can you do?

Pretty much anything to be honest, swimming, walking, team sports, the world is your oyster! Why not put up a net in your back garden for a great way to play several sports? Or if you live on an estate, then why not get together with your neighbours and build a small playground and get your local neighbourhood fit at the same time. If this isn't practical, why not get out with a football and have a good kick around? The aim is to have fun, fun means that you will all enjoy it.

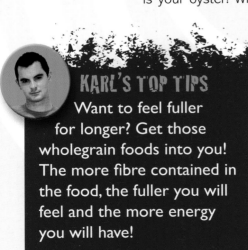

KARL'S TOP TIPS
Want to feel fuller for longer? Get those wholegrain foods into you! The more fibre contained in the food, the fuller you will feel and the more energy you will have!

Hill walking also provides a fantastic way to get fit as a family, as I have mentioned, up the Wicklow hills or anywhere local to you with a packed lunch is a beautiful way to spend a crisp winter's morning and introduce your children to the benefits of exercise and fresh air, showing them that family

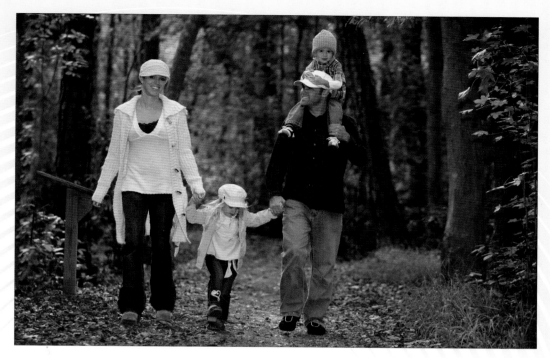

time isn't just about sitting around the TV with a big pizza. It is about creating a healthy environment for you and your family. Remember that you are creating habits that will stay with your child for a lifetime!

By changing your family's exercise habits, improving your food (by cutting out the white refined carbohydrates, such as white rice, white pasta and white bread, as well as the sugar-packed foods), you will set positive affirmations that your children will take into their future.

Another topical but great idea is weighing your child. Do you know how much your child weighs? I would suggest that you weigh your child once every 6 months. To see if they are at a good weight, simply check out the weight/height list for children that was provided by Dr Donal O'Shea for RTÉ's *Operation Transformation* on www.rte.ie/ot.

Children will keep the habits they learn when they are young, don't you think that it is important that you instil exercise as a lifetime habit for them? I think that since the Celtic tiger economy, parents have lost sight of the fact that their children need to come first, rather than the parties and nights out – or even working all the hours that there are in the day. It's so easy to pass the blame, but, guess what – you are the parent, it's your responsibility.

Childhood obesity is one of my passions, it was the subject of my first-class honours thesis in my degree in UCD. Children now suffer from weight-related issues, type 2 diabetes, sleep apnoea, cholesterol and several other conditions, and this state of affairs is only going to get worse unless we stop it. People power is the way to solve the childhood obesity epidemic, so come on people, let's solve this crisis and instil health in our children – they are the future.

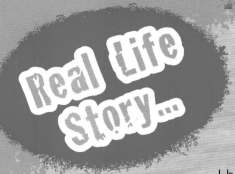

Real Life Story...

It's almost a year to the day since I stood on the scales and concluded that I could not gain another ounce or allow the dial on the scales to climb another notch. I felt awful, I looked terrible and my clothes did not fit. I was overweight.

I had always been conscious of my health; I knew the importance of exercise and a balanced diet for my physical and mental well being. Yet, despite this, I found myself going to the gym less and less often and selecting the quick fixes rather than the healthy options when it came to food.

I didn't fall into this trap deliberately. My job was getting busier and I had more and more commitments in the evenings and weekends. I felt my gym membership was like a charitable donation – I paid the monthly subscription, but my feet never crossed the door. What little spare time I had was reserved for catching up with friends and family. Not surprisingly, I felt my clothes begin to shrink; my waistline was expanding.

One Friday evening, I decided something had to change. I had to stop mistreating by body. I sent an e-mail enquiring about personal training sessions – an e-mail that essentially transformed my life.

Since then, I have lost about thirty-five pounds in weight, my shape has changed completely and, with this, has come an enormous increase in my self-confidence.

The road to my success was not smooth. Sometimes, I compare it to a rollercoaster ride; a journey filled with highs, with lows, with anxiety, with anticipation and, of course, with moments when I felt like I was thrown into the air and turned completely upside down.

The physical part of the journey, the diet and the exercise, was probably the easiest. I kept a diary for the first few weeks where I recorded what I ate and how long I spent in the gym. My motto was simple, 'If I'm too ashamed to write it down, then I shouldn't eat it.' If I skipped the gym, I had to write down why. All of a sudden, an appointment with *Desperate Housewives* no longer seemed like a valid excuse!

I exercised five to six times a week. This was probably excessive, but I reckoned that, the more I did, the easier it would get and the less muscle pain I would suffer after a workout.

There were days when I felt tempted to drive past the gym, but I forced myself to go. As a compromise I would do a short workout on the machines that I really enjoyed. Funnily enough, at the end of these sessions, I always came away from the gym feeling really happy with myself. More importantly for me, it meant that I did not break my pattern of going to the gym on the way home from work each evening.

I found the toughest part of my journey was dealing with my emotions. When I looked at myself in the mirror last year, my self-esteem was at an all-time low. I did not know how I would cope if I gained any more weight. I knew I had reached the turning point, but I was anxious about what lay ahead of me and whether or not I would be strong enough to achieve my goals.

For the first few months, I used to sit outside the gym before my weekly training session with a knot in my stomach. A string of questions would go through my mind: *How I had allowed myself to gain so much weight? How was I ever going to lose it? Would I be fit enough to make it through the next hour?*

I was always nervous starting the session but, by the time, I had finished it, I was always motivated and looking forward to working even harder the following week.

My greatest fear was of not losing the weight I needed and how others would judge me for this. Who would I be letting down – my friends, my family or, most significantly for me, my trainer? Strangely, I never really considered that I would be letting myself down. To deal with this fear, I only included one other person in the initial stages of my journey – my trainer. I felt that if people didn't know about what I was trying to do, then I couldn't disappoint them. This was probably a bit extreme – a little bit of support from close friends can be good, otherwise it can be a very lonely road to travel along.

My journey is not over. I still get embarrassed about the fact that I needed to lose so much weight and I feel uneasy talking to people about it. I find it difficult to congratulate myself and to reward myself for reaching my mile stones.

For anybody trying to achieve a similar goal, I would say be honest with yourself and admit you have to lose weight, be fair to your body and treat it as it deserves to be treated, be good to yourself and reward yourself along the way. There's nothing quite like the feeling of buying a new pair of skinny jeans!

How hard should you push yourself?

Every year, there are people who burn out after a few weeks of training having pushed themselves too hard, too quickly. There are two ways to avoid this, thus ensuring that you reach your goals safely and avoid the dreaded burnout.

The first method is called RPE, or rate of perceived exertion. What this means is that you learn to measure and judge your effort according to five distinct levels. This is a way to measure your effort that works – and it's free, which is always good. Most of your sessions should be either moderate or hard in order for you to get the best results. If you're going out for a walk and find it easy, then chances you aren't getting the best workout for your time. There are many different versions of this system (some more complicated than others) but here is my simple version.

The five levels are as follows.

Level	Exertion	Example
1	Very Easy	Sitting
2	Easy	Walking
3	Moderate	Jogging
4	Hard	Running
5	Very Hard	Sprinting

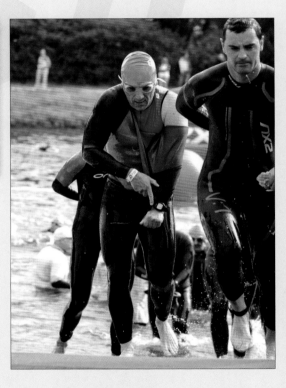

This method works very well but if you are looking to take your training to the next level, then I recommend that you buy a heart-rate monitor watch. This is the second method for measuring your work rate to ensure you avoid burnout. These are the ultimate in technology, giving you all the information you will need to ensure that you are getting the best workout possible. When you work out, your heart pumps faster – the harder you work, the faster your heart beats. A heart-rate monitor will measure this speed.

'Why is this important?' I hear you ask. Your body will burn different fuel depending on your heart rate. If you are looking to burn fat from your body, then there is a heart rate that will do this, if you just want to get fit, there is a heart rate that will do this too. There are 5 different heart-rate zones, and each zone burns a different fuel. Let's take a look at the zones in more detail.

Zone	Heart rate	% of max heart rate	Fuel
1		50-60	Carbs/Protein/Fat
2		60-70	Carbs/Fat
3		70-80	Fat
4		80-90	Carbs/Protein/Fat
5		90-100	Protein

You will notice that I have left the heart-rate box empty, that's because I am going to show you how to calculate your own zones and I want you to insert your heart zones into the heart-rate box. Ready to go?

There are many different ways to do this, but I always find the following method the best, and the simplest, to follow. While it is not exact, it is close enough to give you a good guideline for your workouts.

Subtract your age from 220. This will give you your maximum heart rate. Now work out your zones from the percentages in each zone.

Here is my own example:

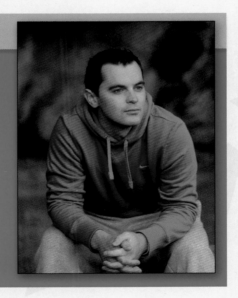

I am 28 – therefore my maximum heart rate is 192.

220-28 = 192

ZONE 1 = 95-114 50-60%

ZONE 2 = 114-133 60-70%

ZONE 3 = 133-152 70-80%

ZONE 4 = 152-171 80-90%

ZONE 5 = 171-192 90-100%

How did you get on?

You should now know your heart-rate zones, so that the next time you are working out, you will be able to monitor how hard you are working. You can do this in two ways: measuring your pulse or by buying a heart-rate monitor watch, which can vary from being simple to incredibly complicated, giving you a lot of different information. Unless you're a serious athlete, simple is the way to go.

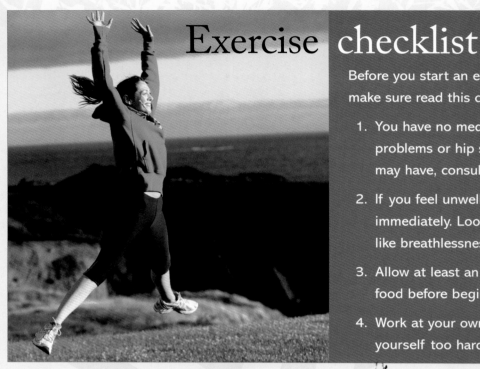

Exercise checklist

Before you start an exercise programme make sure read this checklist.

1. You have no medical problems, back problems or hip soreness. If you feel you may have, consult your GP.

2. If you feel unwell at any stage, stop immediately. Look out for signs of stress like breathlessness or feeling dizzy.

3. Allow at least an hour-and-a-half after food before beginning your routine.

4. Work at your own pace. Don't push yourself too hard.

KARL'S PULSE-TAKING TIP

Take your index and middle finger and place them under the right side of your jaw, close to your neck. Count the number of beats for 15 seconds and multiply by 4 for your heart rate and compare to what you want it to be from the chart.

The watch works by placing a strap around your chest, which sends the information to the watch on your wrist. It is important to point out that this is a very simple method of calculating your heart rate, there are several factors that can affect your heart rate but this simple way of measuring it will give you a pretty accurate result. It is important to note that training in pretty much all of the top three zones will burn fat, but the best zone, from my experience, is certainly zone 3.

Muscle pain and how to recover faster

When you start exercising, there is a chance that you are going to be in pain to some degree. If you start gradually and build your fitness up steadily, you will be fine, but exercise too much too soon and there will be pain, plenty of it! But what causes this pain?

Your muscles are made up of interconnected fibres. When you train, you stretch and cause minute tears in the fibres, leading to the burning sensation that you feel. In the days after training, you will more than likely get what is called DOMS – delayed onset muscle soreness – as your muscles repair and grow back together, stronger and firmer. This normally occurs on the second day after your workout, it is not a sign of injury or anything serious, it is simply your body's reaction to the fact that it is now doing something that it isn't used to doing. Over the course of several weeks, your body will adapt to the training and you will begin to recover faster from your workouts, leading to far less pain. Our bodies are incredible and adapt rapidly to the new strains and stresses that we place on it.

Now you know what happens when you train, what can you do to prevent muscle soreness?

▸ Cool down/stretch at the end of your workout. At the end of every workout aim to cool down with some simple stretching.

▸ Call into your local chemist and buy some Epsom salts. Place 1 or 2 cupfuls into a nice hot bath and sit back and relax for 30 minutes. The salts will diffuse into your muscles and relax them like nothing else!

▸ If your muscles are sore during the day, then apply some Deep Heat gel. Although this may smell quite strongly, it will heat up and relax your sore aches and pains very quickly.

▸ For those of you are brave, try some cold therapy to loosen the body out. Straight after a session jump into an ice-cold bath or into the sea for 5 to 10 minutes for super fast recovery.

▸ If the stiffness persists for longer than 2 days then don't skip your workout. Take it easy at your next session and after 5 or 10 minutes of that session, your body will loosen up nicely and you will forget that you ever had any pain.

Types of exercise

There are three different types of exercise that I am going to look at over the coming pages.

- **Cardiovascular:** Cardiovascular exercise comes in any form basically that works the lungs, it is the ability of your heart, lungs and organs to consume, transport and utilise oxygen. Everything from hill walking to running will provide you with a great workout. Your whole body is exercised when you do any form of cardiovascular workout.

- **Resistance:** Resistance training is a form of strength training in which each effort is performed against a specific opposing force generated by resistance (i.e. resistance to being pushed, squeezed, stretched or bent). Exercises are isotonic if a body part is moving against the force. Exercises are isometric if a body part is holding still against the force. Resistance exercise is used to develop the strength and size of skeletal muscles. These workouts can be done in gyms or pretty much anywhere.

Some common words you may hear

Reps

A rep is, very simply, a movement, one rep equals one movement of the exercise. Different numbers of reps are designed to do different things. Lower reps are generally designed to build muscle and higher reps are designed to tone muscles. In this book, you will see that I only use high reps as this is the method that, in my opinion, will give the best results.

Sets

A set is simply the number of times you do a number of reps. For example, I might ask you to do 3 sets of 20 reps. This means that you should do 20 reps 3 times. Different training plans use a different numbers of sets — normally from 3 to 10. In the following pages, you will see that I generally recommend 3 sets as I find this optimal for toning the body.

Endorphins

Endorphins are compounds released from the pituitary gland in the brain during exercise. These are the reason that you feel so good after exercise. They are called the happy hormone and are one of the best natural ways to fight off bad moods and depression. The best way to get this is prolonged exercise of 30 minutes or more. What better way to get a natural high! These compounds will not only improve your mood, they will also improve your concentration levels, your productivity levels, your relationships and you will feel less hungry too. All of a sudden, life will seem better, easier and you will relish the challenges ahead. This all comes from the fantastic endorphin.

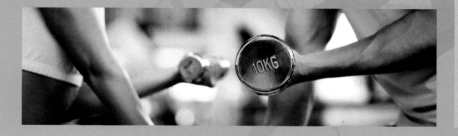

Resistance exercise will:

- Decrease stomach fat.
- Reduce stress.
- Reduce the risk of cardiovascular disease.
- Release endorphins.
- Burn more calories.
- Keep you feeling young.
- Increase your bone density.
- Make you sleep better.
- Help you live longer.
- Help you fight depression.
- Get better results, faster.

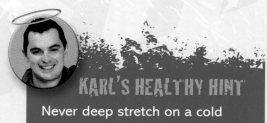

▸ **Flexibilty:** Flexibility workouts refer to a set of exercises that boost our flexibility. These mainly involve stretching exercises. Workouts such as yoga, Pilates and tai chi are all based around flexibility. It is essential to stretch after each workout to ensure that your muscles don't get tight and cause you pain. Stretching also reduces the chances of you tearing a muscle. The tighter the muscle is, the higher the likelihood that you may get injured.

Posture

Your posture is one of the key components in safe and effective exercise practice. Put simply, posture is the position of your spine in relation to your body. A good posture will be similar to the diagram below.

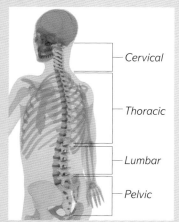

Cervical

Thoracic

Lumbar

Pelvic

All too often, I see people exercising with poor posture, with their backs arched too much or with very rounded shoulders. As you age, your posture worsens as your muscles get weaker, you need to exercise to keep your body straight. Men can also be the worst offenders of this, especially in the gym environment. This is all down to the male ego. In striving to lift heavier and heavier weights, posture becomes very poor, which can lead to back problems and even back damage. For safe and effective exercise, posture is key.

Cardiovascular fitness

This refers to the ability of your heart, lungs and organs to consume, transport and utilise oxygen. If you get out of breath when walking up the stairs, then your lungs and heart aren't in great shape — your cardiovascular fitness is low. Therefore, you need to get more activity into your day to improve your fitness levels.

Not only is posture key for exercise, it is also key for visual improvements. With poor posture your shoulders look narrower, you develop a pot belly and your chest naturally becomes softer and looks worse. Pull those shoulders back, stand tall and instantly you will look better, your stomach will flatten, your arms and shoulders will look better too. Try it the next time you look in the mirror for yourself and you will be amazed by the results.

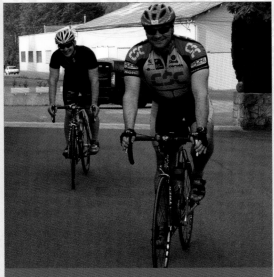

How long should you spend training

Some people think that 30 minutes is enough exercise for 1 session, some think that it should be an hour and a half. In my opinion, an hour is long enough to get the best workout and to make it part of your life. This should include your warm up, workout and cool down. If you are spending longer in the gym, I think that you're spending too long, taking too long between sets and spending too much time looking in the mirror! In order to fit exercise into your life on a long-term basis, balance is key!

Three hours a week should be easy to fit into anyone's schedule. Obviously, if you are training for a marathon or other events, you will need to spend more time but, generally, 1 hour per session is plenty of time.

Sports

The key to keeping healthy for life is finding a sport that you enjoy. If you hate running, chances are that you won't keep up running for very long. If you enjoy something, then you will find it easier to keep up and you will get more benefits from it as it's fun! But don't be afraid to try new sports either. Every year, I aim to try at least one new sport, after all, if you don't try it then how will you know if you will like it or not? The older we get, the more barriers we build up around us, and the more reluctant we become to try something new. So go on give it a try, you might just find a new sport that you never thought you would enjoy! Here a just a few of my favourites.

Walking

Here is one of the biggest secrets in the fitness industry, that more and more people are beginning to realise... walking is one of the best ways to get fit! Now I have read articles by other trainers who would knock this but, believe you me, walking – not strolling but fast walking – is one of the most nationally accessible ways to get fit. All you need is a pair of runners and some road and out you go, simple as that! It is easy to do, gives you incredible health benefits and anyone of any age can do it anywhere in the country.

Why fast walking works wonders.

▸ It strengthens the cardiovascular system.

▸ It tones muscles.

▸ It increases flexibility.

▸ It reduces stress.

▸ It lowers fat.

▸ It works your legs and bum.

▸ It helps reduce cellulite.

Now by walking, I don't mean strolling round the house, I am talking about doing an average of 4 miles an hour,

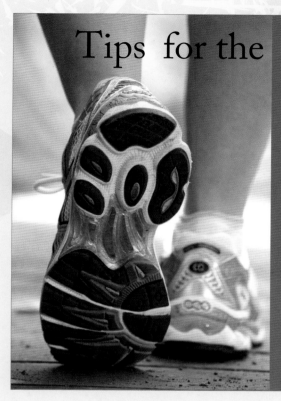

Tips for the ultimate walk workout

▷ Choose a route you enjoy and one that's not too far from your home (the park, beach, etc.).

▷ Measure the distance in a car, 4 miles is optimum.

▷ Get a walking buddy. You can motivate each other to get out!

▷ Walk heel to toe. This helps to prevent knee and back strain.

▷ Get a good pair of runners or walking shoes, these will help prevent injuries — and sore feet. Ideally, change your runners every 3 months if you are doing a lot of exercise

▷ Change your stride every 10 to 15 minutes, this will help prevent soreness and stiffness in your joints.

▷ Try to change your route on a weekly basis.

at a brisk pace! This works out at walking that magic 15-minute mile, which is the optimum to get the best health benefits! If you find this pace too fast, then just walk at whatever pace you feel comfortable at and aim to build up your pace. And most important of all — HAVE FUN!

If you can, grab a friend and get them to come out with you, or set up a walking group — friends are great for motivation and you can get fit together!

If you are looking for some more motivation then why not get a pedometer and measure your steps in a day, ideally you should be looking to get 10,000 steps a day in on a normal day, pedometers can be purchased in most sports shops and just clip onto your belt.

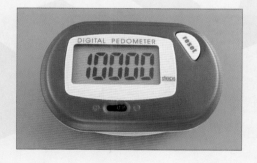

It is best to map out a course for yourself, so that you know where you are going before you set out. A good way to do this is to measure the route in your car. An even easier method to measure your route is to use the internet. There is an amazing website called www.mapmyrun.com which is a free website that will let you track your route using your mouse and will give you all the feedback that you need in terms of distance and elevation.

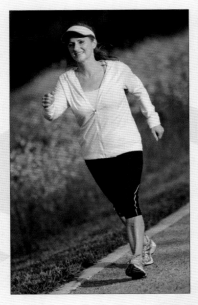

Why is walking so good:

▸ It's free!

▸ 1 hour of brisk walking burns 400-500 calories.

▸ It places a minimal amount of stress on the body. A walker's foot receives 1 to 1.5 times the body weight per stride, compared to running which places 3 to 4 times the body weight with each stride.

▸ It's easy and accessible to all.

▸ There is no age limit on who can walk.

▸ You will have more energy than ever before, guaranteed.

For those of you who are finding walking too easy, you can make these simple adaptations to make things a little tougher for yourself.

▸ **Stride walking.** Simply bring light hand weights along with you and stride your arms by your side.

▸ **Increase your speed.** Aim for 5 mph rather than 4 mph.

▸ **Stair climbing.** If you have access to a building with lots of stairs then you have no excuse – 15 to 20 minutes of climbing stairs is one of the greatest cardiovascular exercises as well. If you are walking outside and there are steps along your route, use these to enhance your workout.

Remember the measurements that we discussed in the introduction section? Try to use the perceived rate of exertion when you are walking to ensure that you are getting the best workout possible!

Karl's Tips for Success

If at first you don't succeed, try try again. Make a pact that you will persist at all costs until you do indeed succeed!

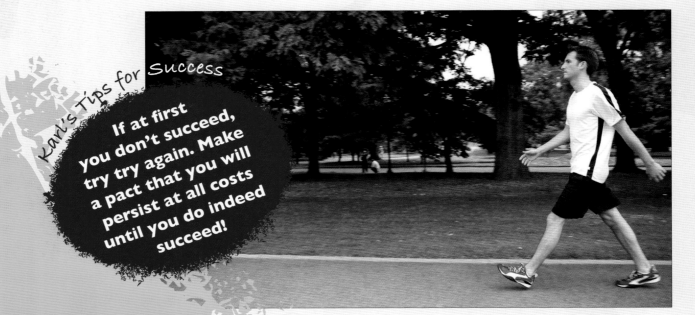

Real Results

Running

The first question I always ask people when we discuss running is this: Are you running for fun or because you think it will help you become slim?

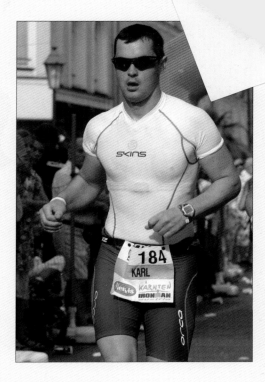

Think about it for a minute yourself, why do you run? In my opinion, you need to run for fun and enjoyment first! Like any form of exercise, for it to last, you must enjoy it otherwise you may do it for a few weeks but it won't last long term. Running and fast walking have very similar benefits, so only run if you truly want to. When I began to turn my life around and get fit, running was the tool that I used. I revelled in the post-run feeling, the sense of freedom and the sense of fitness too. I began running half marathons, then marathons and recently ultra marathons. I have made all the mistakes and am going to tell you about them – so that you won't make them too.

You don't need much to get started but the most important thing is a pair of runners.

Take a look at the sole of your runners, if they are unevenly worn on one side then you need a new pair. For me, Asics are the best brand on the market, especially the Gel Kayano's. Nike and Adidas are catching up fast but I will always be an Asics man. They are expensive but they are well worth it. When buying your runners, you should ask to have a gait analysis done which is available in all Lifestyle Sports stores around the country. This will mean that you get the best runner suited to your foot.

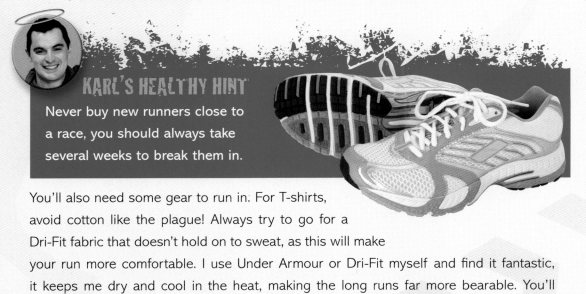

KARL'S HEALTHY HINT

Never buy new runners close to a race, you should always take several weeks to break them in.

You'll also need some gear to run in. For T-shirts, avoid cotton like the plague! Always try to go for a Dri-Fit fabric that doesn't hold on to sweat, as this will make your run more comfortable. I use Under Armour or Dri-Fit myself and find it fantastic, it keeps me dry and cool in the heat, making the long runs far more bearable. You'll also need a rain jacket should be light and wind/water proof. The lighter the better as you don't want to be wearing heavy clothing. We all know that the Irish weather is temperamental at the best of times, so always be prepared!

Next are some running tights – no matter how embarrassing they may look, when you get into them, you'll never go back! They not only keep you warm but they help to keep the muscles protected too and can also prevent chafing. Another essential investment is a good pair of socks. These will make you feel more comfortable while running, prevent blisters and also will dry quickly when they get wet. They will have more material in the areas of the foot that you need extra support. There are so many brands on the market and any good sports store will have a big selection. You may not think that socks would make much of a difference but, I promise you, they do. Try out a new pair the next time that you are in your local Lifestyle Sports store.

 Did You Know?

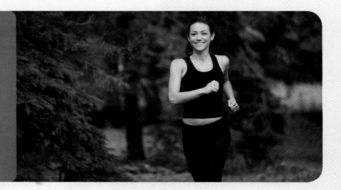

You can help prevent blisters or chafing using Vaseline. A small amount of Vaseline on your feet will help to prevent blisters and on the inside of the legs, armpits and nipples will help to prevent chafing.

You have the gear now and are ready to start running, what next? If you are new to running, then patience will be key. You need to start off slow and build yourself up. Begin by testing yourself, start running and see how long you last. Then you need to begin your training. A good base programme will see you do 2 or 3 short runs and 1 long run per week. If you need to walk at the beginning then, don't stress about it, the fitter you get the less you will walk. Every 2 or 3 weeks, you should be increasing you distance slowly. So for example, if your first week runs were 4 km and 6 km at the weekend, then the next step up should be 5 km and 8 km, and so on.

The quickest way to improve your running fitness is interval training. I will be talking about this in more detail on page 130 but, basically, it means that you should be training using 2 speeds – one easy and the second faster. You vary the intervals so that you jog/walk slowly for 5 minutes and run fast for 5 minutes, then back to slow again. As you get fitter you simply reduce the slow interval and increase the fast interval.

The next important factor to look at is the terrain that you are running on. If you continue to just run on a flat surface, then your body will adapt to that. You need to keep changing the surface from hills to cross country and back to flat again. You will find that your fitness will continue to increase in leaps and bounds if you vary your training like this.

Real Results

Below are four simple interval running programmes designed to get you running.

Programme	Slow	Fast	Sets
1	5 minute walk	3 minute jog	5
2	5 minute walk	5 minute jog	6
3	5 minute walk	8 minute jog	4
4	5 minute walk	10 minute jog	4

As your fitness improves, why not register for a race? You will find that you will always race faster than you will train so it is a great way of pushing yourself that little bit harder and it gives you a great goal. The running plans on pages 100–103 will give you detailed plans that will deliver great results in whatever distance race you choose to do.

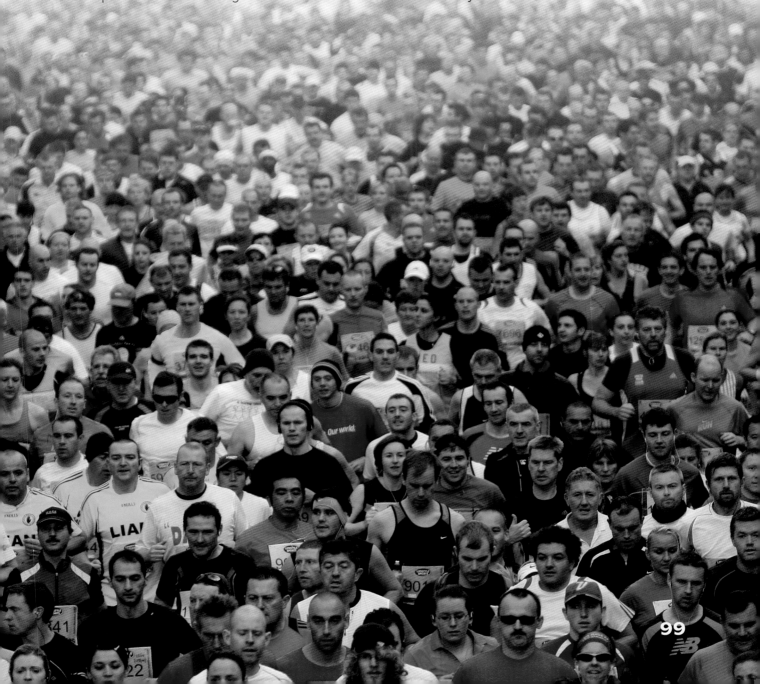

TRAINING PLANS

Marathon walking plan

This plan is fantastic for anyone who would love to walk the marathon and is built on just 3 sessions per week over the course of 19 weeks.

Week	Session 1	Session 2	Session 3
1	4 miles	2 miles	6 miles
2	4 miles	2 miles	6 miles
3	4 miles	2 miles	6 miles
4	5 miles	3 miles	8 miles
5	5 miles	3 miles	8 miles
6	5 miles	4 miles	10 miles
7	4 miles	4 miles	10 miles
8	4 miles	4 miles	10 miles
9	6 miles	4 miles	10 miles
10	6 miles	4 miles	12 miles
11	4 miles	4 miles	12 miles
12	4 miles	4 miles	14 miles
13	4 miles	4 miles	14 miles
14	6 miles	4 miles	16 miles
15	4 miles	4 miles	16 miles
16	4 miles	4 miles	18 miles
17	Rest	2 miles	20 miles
18	Rest	2 miles	20 miles
19	4 miles	Rest	Marathon

5-km run plan

This plan is ideal for anyone looking to do their first 5-km race!
Use Monday and Friday as rest days.

Week	Tuesday	Wednesday	Thursday	Saturday	Sunday
1	1.5 mile run	1 hour gym cardio	1.5 mile run	2 mile run	30 minute run easy
2	2 mile run	1 hour gym cardio	1 mile run	2.5 mile run	30 minute run easy
3	2 mile run	1 hour gym cardio	1.5 mile run	2.5 mile run	30 minute run easy
4	2.5 mile run	1 hour gym cardio	1.5 mile run	3 mile run	35-40 minute run easy
5	3 mile run	1 hour gym cardio	1.5 mile run	3.5 mile run	35-40 minute run easy
6	3.5 mile run	1 hour gym cardio	1.5 mile run	4 mile run	35-40 minute run easy
7	3 mile run	1 hour gym cardio	1.5 mile run (race pace)	4 mile run	40 minute run easy
8	3 mile run	Rest	2 mile run	Rest	Race

10-km run plan

Every fancy a 10-km run? Well, here is the best training plan for
you! Use Tuesdays, Thursdays and Saturdays as rest days.

Week	Monday	Wednesday	Friday	Sunday	Total
1	2 miles	4 miles	3 miles	3 miles	12 miles
2	2 miles	4 miles	2 miles	4 miles	12 miles
3	2 miles	3 miles	2 miles	5 miles	12 miles
4	2 miles	4 miles	2 miles	5 miles	13 miles
5	2 miles	6 miles	2 miles	4 miles	14 miles
6	2 miles	2 miles	2 miles	Race	6 miles

Half-marathon training plan

You have decided to do a half-marathon but don't know where to start, well here is the plan for you.

Week	Monday	Tuesday	Wednesday	Thursday	Friday	Saturday	Sunday
1	Rest	2 miles	Rest	2.5 miles	Rest	3 miles	2 miles easy
2	Rest	2 miles	Rest	3 miles	Rest	4 miles	2.5 miles easy
3	Rest	2.5 miles	1 hour gym	3 miles	Rest	5 miles	2 miles easy
4	Rest	3 miles	1 hour gym	4 miles	Rest	6 miles	3 miles easy
5	Rest	3 miles	1 hour gym	3 miles	Rest	7 miles	3 miles easy
6	Rest	4 miles	1 hour gym	4 miles	Rest	8 miles	3 miles easy
7	Rest	4 miles	1 hour gym	4 miles	rest	9 miles	3 miles easy
8	Rest	4 miles	Gym	3 miles	Rest	10 miles	3 miles easy
9	Rest	5 miles	1 hour gym	4 miles	Rest	11 miles	Rest
10	3 miles easy	4 miles	Rest	3 miles	Rest	12 miles	3 miles easy
11	Rest	2 miles	Rest	3 miles	Rest	5 miles	2.5 miles easy
12	Rest	2 miles	20 minutes	Rest	20 minutes	Race	Rest

Sub-five-hour marathon training plan

A great plan for the beginner marathon runner.

Week	Monday	Tuesday	Wednesday	Thursday	Friday	Saturday	Sunday
1	3 miles	Rest	3 miles	3 miles	Rest	3 miles	4 miles
2	3 miles	Rest	3 miles	3 miles	Rest	3 miles	4 miles
3	3 miles	Rest	3 miles	3 miles	Rest	3 miles	4 miles
4	3 miles	Rest	3 miles	3 miles	Rest	3 miles	4 miles
5	4 miles	Rest	5 miles	6 miles	Rest	6 miles	7 miles
6	4 miles	Rest	5 miles	6 miles	Rest	6 miles	7 miles
7	4 miles	Rest	5 miles	6 miles	Rest	6 miles	7 miles
8	4 miles	Rest	5 miles	6 miles	Rest	6 miles	7 miles
9	6 miles	Rest	6 miles	5 miles	Rest	6 miles	10 miles
10	6 miles	Rest	6 miles	5 miles	Rest	6 miles	10 miles
11	6 miles	Rest	6 miles	6 miles	Rest	6 miles	12 miles
12	6 miles	Rest	6 miles	6 miles	Rest	6 miles	12 miles
13	6 miles	Rest	6 miles	6 miles	Rest	6 miles	14 miles
14	6 miles	Rest	6 miles	6 miles	Rest	6 miles	14 miles
15	6 miles	Rest	6 miles	6 miles	Rest	6 miles	16 miles
16	6 miles	Rest	6 miles	6 miles	Rest	6 miles	16 miles
17	6 miles	6 miles	6 miles	6 miles	Rest	6 miles	18 miles
18	6 miles	6 miles	6 miles	6 miles	Rest	6 miles	18 miles
19	6 miles	6 miles	6 miles	6 miles	Rest	6 miles	14 miles
20	6 miles	6 miles	6 miles	6 miles	Rest	6 miles	14 miles
21	4 miles	2 miles	3 miles	3 miles	2 miles	Rest	Marathon

Sub-four-hour marathon training plan

The interval sessions on Tuesdays and Thursdays are basically normal pace for 2 minutes then sprint for 2 minutes.

Week	Monday	Tuesday	Wednesday	Thursday	Friday	Saturday	Sunday
1	6 miles	Rest	6 miles	6 miles	Rest	6 miles	8 miles
2	6 miles	Rest	6 miles	6 miles	Rest	6 miles	8 miles
3	6 miles	Rest	6 miles	6 miles	Rest	6 miles	8 miles
4	6 miles	Rest	6 miles	6 miles	Rest	6 miles	8 miles
5	8 miles	Rest	8 miles	6 miles interval	Rest	6 miles	10 miles
6	8 miles	Rest	8 miles	6 miles interval	Rest	6 miles	10 miles
7	8 miles	Rest	8 miles	6 miles interval	Rest	6 miles	10 miles
8	8 miles	Rest	8 miles	6 miles interval	Rest	6 miles	10 miles
9	8 miles	6 miles interval	7 miles	8 miles interval	Rest	6 miles	14 miles
10	8 miles	6 miles interval	7 miles	8 miles interval	Rest	6 miles	14 miles
11	8 miles	8 miles interval	7 miles	8 miles interval	Rest	6 miles	16 miles
12	8 miles	8 miles interval	7 miles	8 miles interval	Rest	6 miles	16 miles
13	8 miles	10 miles interval	7 miles	10 miles interval	Rest	6 miles	18 miles
14	8 miles	10 miles interval	7 miles	10 miles interval	Rest	6 miles	18 miles
15	8 miles	10 miles interval	8 miles	10 miles interval	Rest	6 miles	20 miles
16	8 miles	10 miles interval	8 miles	10 miles interval	Rest	6 miles	20 miles
17	8 miles	10 miles interval	8 miles	10 miles interval	Rest	6 miles	20 miles
18	8 miles	10 miles interval	8 miles	10 miles interval	Rest	6 miles	20 miles
19	8 miles	10 miles interval	8 miles	10 miles interval	Rest	6 miles	18 miles
20	8 miles	10 miles interval	8 miles	10 miles interval	Rest	6 miles	18 miles
21	5 miles	4 miles interval	5 miles	3 miles	2 miles	2 miles	Marathon

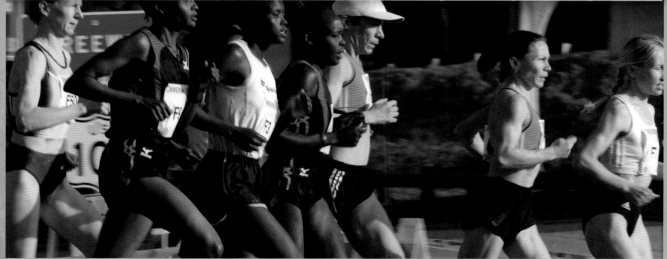

Swimming

Swimming provides you with an amazing way to get fit, without pounding your joints. No matter what your level of fitness is, you will be able to challenge yourself and get your lungs pumping. There are more swimming pools than ever before around the country, so why not get out there and make use of

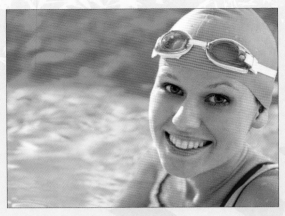

them? If you find that walking or running is giving you sore joints, then try swimming and you will see that you can get an equally good workout from an exercise that doesn't hurt your joints at all.

Every muscle group within your body gets a great workout when you swim – from your calves to your shoulders, your neck to your waist – but there are certain tips that will ensure you get the best workout from your time in the pool.

Swimming is such a simple sport to get involved in. You need togs, and, no, it doesn't have to be the cringe worthy Speedos for the guys, you can get boxer short type gear such as the Speedo endurance range. After this, you need a good set of anti-fog goggles, which are inexpensive. Just get yourself a hat and off you go. For less than €20 you can be in the pool getting fit!

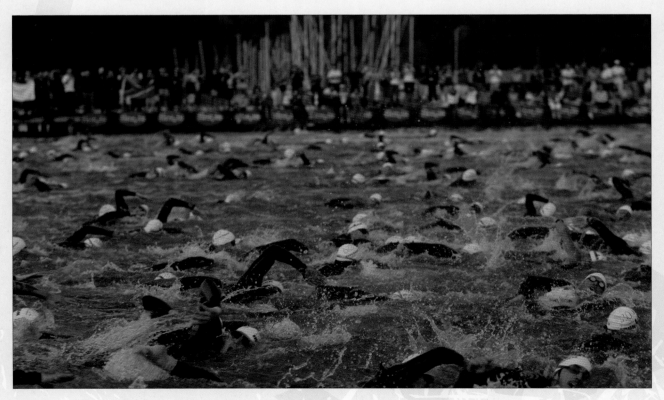

Often, one of the elements that scares people from entering the pool is the people who are flying up and down the lanes – but lane swimmers swim at different paces. In your pool, you will normally find fast and slow lanes. There will also be an area of the pool that will be for beginner swimmers too. So when you walk out to the pool, just look at the swimmers and see which group suits your pace. Normally, the faster lanes will be in the centre of the pool and the slower lanes towards the sides.

There is some etiquette, however. One side will be for swimming up and one for swimming down (not in the middle like the man who was in my lane a few weeks ago). If you get tired, then simply move to the side when you get to one end, it's as simple as that. By observing the lanes, you will feel much more comfortable in the pool, swimming with people that are a similar pace to you.

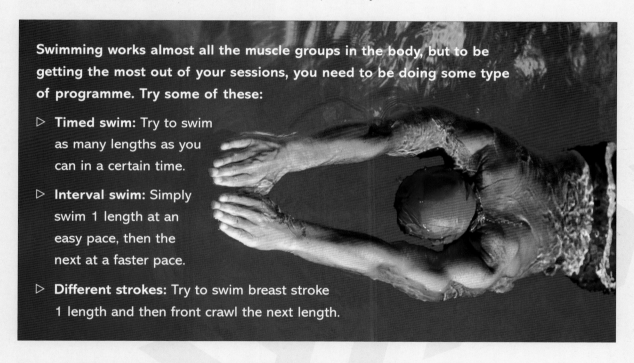

Swimming works almost all the muscle groups in the body, but to be getting the most out of your sessions, you need to be doing some type of programme. Try some of these:

▷ **Timed swim:** Try to swim as many lengths as you can in a certain time.

▷ **Interval swim:** Simply swim 1 length at an easy pace, then the next at a faster pace.

▷ **Different strokes:** Try to swim breast stroke 1 length and then front crawl the next length.

Sometimes, people fail to see results from swimming and there is, generally, one reason for this. By getting into the pool for a swim and just paddling a few lengths, you will see some benefits, but not very many. This is similar to strolling instead of walking. You need to have a plan of action when you get into a pool and the simple programmes above will give you great benefits, such as toned arms, a firmer waist and better aerobic fitness levels.

Cycling

The whole country is on a cycling buzz at the moment with the introduction of the bike-to-work scheme from the government, there are more and more cycle lanes being built and people of all ages are availing of the scheme.

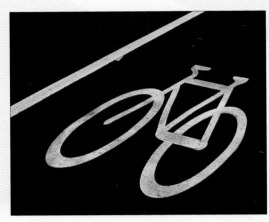

A fantastic form of exercise, cycling works all the major muscle groups, even your upper body which may surprise some people. So let's break it down, you want to start cycling so what do you need?

A bike, obviously! The type of bike depends on your need.

A racing bike is faster and lighter but less stable as the tyres are very thin.

Mountain bikes however are heavier, with thick tyres. They are far more stable on the road but you will need to peddle harder to get up those hills.

You can also get hybrid bikes that are a cross between the two, lighter that a mountain bike with thicker tires than a racer. For people who want to commute, these are probably the best option.

When you are buying your bike, you should be fitted properly by the shop. This includes saddle height and brand of bike. Different bike brands have different build structures. So ensure that the shop assistant picks the right one for you. You will be spending a lot of time on your saddle, so getting a bike fit is really important, this bike won't be gathering dust in the shed!

Type of bike	Weight	Tyres	Tips
Mountain	Heavy	Thick	Great if you live somewhere with bad roads
Hybrid	Average	Average	Great for town/commuting
Racer	Light	Thin	Can be uncomfortable for commuting

Next, you need some essentials for your bike. The first is a puncture repair kit, as well as a small pump. These can be carried in a saddle bag under your saddle, believe me punctures are really easy to fix! The other thing you need are mud guards, these clip on to the bike and will keep you clean and dry so that you don't arrive into work covered in mud. And don't forget your lights! If you haven't got lights then you can't be seen by motorists.

Obviously you need a helmet. If you don't have a helmet, then you shouldn't be allowed to have a bike. If you fall off without a helmet, you risk getting a serious – maybe even fatal – injury! I myself have had one big fall where I went over the top of the bike, if I hadn't been wearing a helmet, I wouldn't be here today writing this book, so forget about fashion and just buy a helmet!

You are nearly there, all you need now is the proper clothing. I am afraid that those Lycra cycling shorts do actually have a purpose. They have in-built padding that help prevent the pain of spending too long in the saddle. The good news is that there are more normal-looking shorts on the market that have the padding without the embarrassing-looking Lycra. If you are just commuting, then get yourself some water proofs, they will just fit over your regular clothes and keep you dry. Cycling provides a great way to get fit and to get you to work in no time. Unlike running, you won't arrive in work covered in sweat, it is more passive so you won't sweat as much. But you will still get a great cardio workout as well as firm legs, even the arms get a workout.

To help keep yourself safe on a bike, remember to use your hands. Indicate left, right or straight ahead using your hands so that other people will know what you are doing. Cyclists are road users and in my opinion need to communicate too so, remember, use those hands!

You have all the tips, you know what to do, the government is trying to help, the traffic is only going to get worse, and you are only going to spend longer in it. Why not take the giant step and try cycling, you will get a great workout and commute to work at the same time, passing all the people stuck in their cars in the traffic.

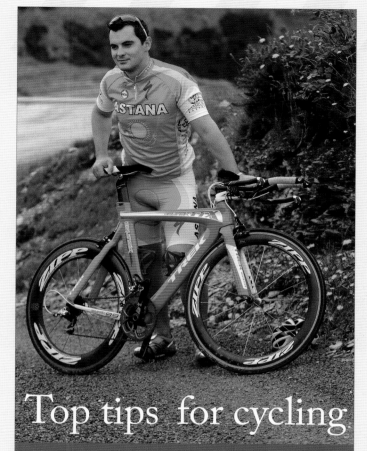

Top tips for cycling

When you're on the road, take note of the following.

We have cycle lanes all over the country. Where possible try to stick to these lanes, they will make life a lot easier and safer on your bike. But watch out for three allies: people, buses and taxi drivers.

▷ **People:** Walkers, runners, prams, rollerbladers! All use the cycle lanes and you are going to have to learn to holler at them. Especially in parks and community areas, so just keep an eye out for people.

▷ **Buses:** In cities, the cycle lanes have bus lanes built in to them too. This means that buses will take up the road including the cycle lane and squash you if you're not careful! Simply let the bus pull in and go around them if possible.

▷ **Taxi drivers:** Similar to buses, taxis can just pull in to cycle lanes at any stage, so be on the lookout for these too.

Mountain biking

If road biking is a little too chilled out for you and you see yourself as an adrenaline junky then look no farther. Mountain biking is a sport that will provide you with all the exhilaration that you need while giving your body a real workout! You will work every muscle in your mind, as well as your body, when you're mountain biking, the terrain changes so quickly that you will need to concentrate every second!

Let's look at what do you need. A bike, helmet and a willingness to challenge yourself, that's it, you're free to go!

In terms of bikes, there are many to choose from: think funky colours, mud guards and suspension forks and your on the right track! Bikes either have no suspension, back suspension, or front and back suspension. It totally depends on what kind of riding your planning to do – but I would recommend that you get at least rear suspension. My own bike is full suspension and I have tested it on the hardest terrain, it takes some serious punishment!

Now that you have your bike, get yourself a good helmet. You all know my opinions on road cycling, but a helmet is even more important in mountain biking. Picture a big muddy ditch, with rocks and thorns and that's where you may end up, so a good helmet is essential. You can also buy protective gloves and body armour too. Although this is not for you purists out there, it is seriously effective if you do come off, you will spare yourself the bruises.

The next item you will need is some cycling padded shorts! If you want to be walking straight the next day, then you are going to need a pair of these. I know they can look embarrassing, and are sometimes not the most flattering, but my goodness are they comfortable. There are normal or Lycra style shorts but the padding is in both and will keep you comfortable.

Here is another great tip: try to buy at least one piece of reflective clothing, sometimes it gets misty and dull on the mountains and you need to be seen! Generally, rain jackets and CamelBaks (hydration backpacks) are the best form to buy, it's all about safety and people being able to see you.

You have bought all the kit, it's gleaming sitting in your kitchen, now its time to get muddy! There are several Coillte trails all over Ireland, Ballinastoe in Wicklow, the amazing Ballyhoura in Limerick/Cork and the new trails in Connemara. These trails have a mixture of mud, man-made tracks, boardwalks, forests, uphill and downhill terrain and make for a safer experience.

Karl's Tips for Success

Check out www.coillte.ie for information on all new mountain bike trails in Ireland.

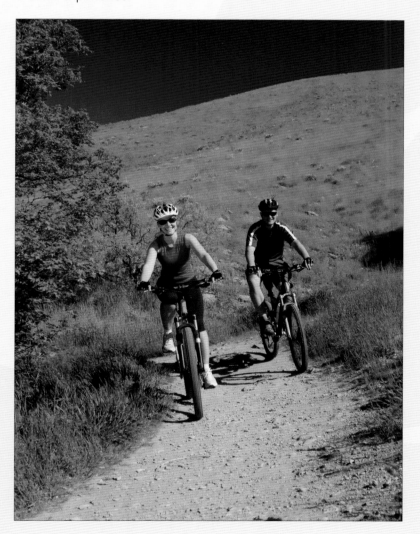

If you are a beginner, I would recommend Ballyhoura in Limerick. There are five super courses, taking from 1 hour to 6 hours, a supervised car park and lovely hot showers afterwards too to wash all that muck away. There is even a bike-wash facility for your new toy so that you're not bringing half of Limerick's muck home with you. The courses are fast, really fast, and will provide you with the biggest adrenaline rush you have had since that rollercoaster all those years ago! Having been there several times, you seen people of all ages in the car park, having a coffee and chatting about their session. Anyone can do this, yes you, as you read this. Why not try it? You won't be left disappointed.

Put aside your fears, dust off your helmet, try the great outdoors for an exhilarating day you won't forget!

Surfing

Think six-packs, think defined shoulders and a narrow waist! That could be you in a few months! There are very few sports that will give your core a better workout than surfing, every motion on the board will engage nearly every muscle in the body. Paddling out to catch a wave will work your shoulders, biceps, back and, yes ladies, those bingo wings! Not only that, but your lungs will get an incredible workout too!

'Talk to me in calories,' I hear you say. One hour of good surf with good waves can burn up to 700 calories! That's equal to two bars of chocolate! As often as possible, I get up to Bundoran with my friend Richie Fitzgerald or to West Cork. Surfing is a fantastic way to relieve the stress from a hard day's work as well as giving the body a great workout!

So how do you start? Get online and find your nearest surfing school, it's that simple. Normally in the region of €35 for a 2-hour lesson, including board and wetsuit (yes you will need one of these, it's kind of cold!). Your instructor will teach you the basics of the board and how to surf. Now we all mightn't be riding the waves straight away, but let go of all those barriers and have some fun, you might just be surprised!

When you have the basics, the sea is yours to surf! The few essentials you'll need are listed below.

Wetsuits vary in price and thickness. The thicker the suit, the warmer it will be, so my advice would be if you want to do this all year round then get a winter wetsuit with a hood (all the heat goes out your head otherwise). I was surfing in Bundoran in -3° at Christmas and couldn't have been warmer, that's how good they are. A simple set of gloves and shoes will ensure that you are lovely and warm. In terms of cost, suits start at around €100 and go up from there. Another essential tip is to try before you buy, when you are in the shop go into the dressing room and try on that wetsuit. Another great tip is to buy your winter wetsuit between April and August as you will get great deals.

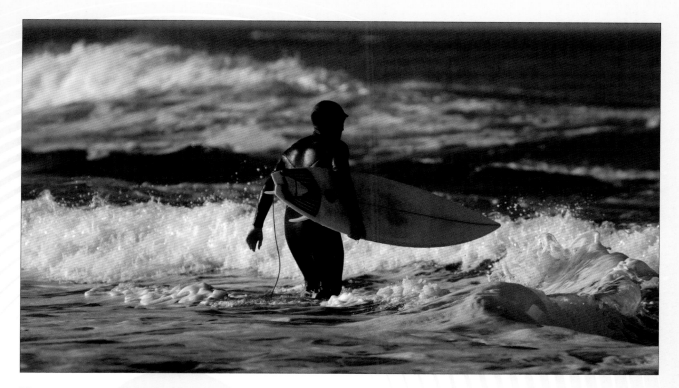

Then you will need a board, your very own tool to surf the waves. When starting, most people go for a long board – 8 ft or 9 ft. These boards are more stable and easier to start on, I know the smaller hand-painted boards look seriously cool, but wait a while until you have mastered the long board. Boards start at around €200 and go upwards from there, most shops will also trade your board in as you get better, so you could even start with a second-hand board.

Surfing is all about practice, when you have the basics learned, off you go! There are clubs all around the country even in Leinster, providing a fantastic way to meet people too. Simply check out www.isasurf.ie for all the details on clubs and how to keep safe while surfing!

Ever wondered the best way to wax your surfboard? Here is what I learned from Richie, he is one of the best surfers in the country so if he doesn't know, who will? You want to wax the board in 2 places, where your feet will be when you're standing. Begin by waxing straight up and down the board, then across the board. Over that patch that you have waxed, apply the wax now in a circular motion. From experience myself, this method provides the best grip on the board. Remember to always wax your board before every surf.

From there, you're ready to ride the waves! It really is that simple. I know it sounds scary, you're sitting reading this thinking there is no way that you could try this, but what have you got to lose? I started surfing a few months ago and on Christmas Day, I had my dad and my brother out, they are now hooked. Here is a sport that can reach all ages, all fitness levels and doesn't cost the earth to start, the only barrier is the one that is stopping you from trying, so go on give it a go.

Tennis

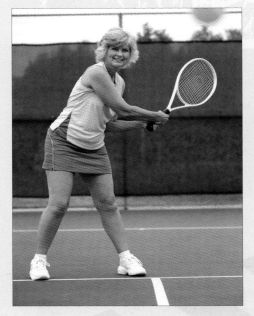

Would you like to burn up to 400 calories per hour? Work your quads, hamstrings, calves, waist, arms and pretty much all the muscles in the upper body, while having fun? Well, guess what? Tennis is the way to go. There are courts vacant all over the country, waiting for someone to play on them, it's out in the fresh air, providing you with a great way to get fit on your doorstep. Literally anyone from 5 to 85 can take part, you can play the game as hard or easy as you want, play for as long as you want and control the intensity level too. Apart from working all your muscles, tennis will give you a great cardiovascular workout.

All you will need are a racket, runners and some tennis balls. Rackets are as cheap as €20 and go upwards from there, some of the more upmarket ones will have shock absorbers built in but generally the cheaper one will do to start with.

Can't remember how the game works? Simple: tennis consists of sets. Each set has 6 games and each game follows the following scoring system 15, 30, 40 and game point. The best of 3 sets wins the match. Sound a little complicated? Trust me, it isn't. When you start playing, you will realise just how easy it is!

One of the main reasons that people are scared of tennis is because the serve is seen as a scary experience! But you don't have to do the big fancy overarm serve if you're not comfortable with it, you can even serve underarm! There really are very few excuses to you not getting on a tennis court, any age, any fitness level, any body type can get out there and play.

Hill walking

The government body in charge of forestry, Coillte, has been busy creating walking routes all over the country, with mile markers, routes and guidelines to show you exactly where to go to get started. They have over 150 routes and that list is growing on a monthly basis. From Cork to Cavan, Wicklow to Waterford there is a route for everybody. There are literally miles and miles of marked trails up and down the country.

So what do you need to get started? The first thing is a pair of walking boots. There are so many brands on the market so there's lots of choice, but make sure you get fitted properly for them. There are 2 main types: low ankle and full boot. A low ankle boot is like a normal runner with a better sole and tougher exterior. These are great for trails without too much heavy terrain or slippery ground. The full boot has a much higher ankle which provides great support, especially when the ground is very mucky. I would recommend a full boot as you will be able to use these all year round when the weather is bad, they are so much safer and you won't regret it.

Try to use the boots for around an hour a day for roughly a week before you go out on your first walk, simply to break them in, this will help prevent blisters when you go out walking the first time. From there, you need to get some socks and not just the ordinary cotton kind! Hill walking puts a much greater stress on your feet so you are going to need some good socks and, without a doubt, thick wool socks are the best. They will make it far more comfortable in those new boots, and deal better with sweat and water that normal socks. Here is another great tip: Before you go out in your new boots, simply rub some Vaseline around your feet and at the back of your foot, to prevent blisters while you're out walking – simple but great!

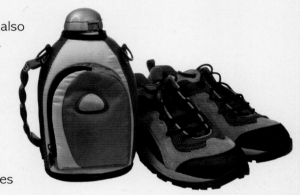

Hill walking provides a fantastic aerobic workout for your lungs, it also provides a challenge every time you go out, by trying to beat your previous time for the walk. The fitter you get, the faster you will get up the hill, simple as that. Hill walking will work your quads (the front of your legs), your hamstrings (the back of your legs) and your calves. It will also work your waist and upper body as you use this part of your body to ascend hills. If you find that you are getting back or shoulder pain, simply buy some walking poles and that will solve the problem!

You have the shoes, the socks and are nearly ready to go! There are two more items that you will need. The first is a good rain jacket. Buy a jacket that is lightweight, windproof and waterproof. The heavier the jacket, the heavier it will feel when you're 500 feet up a mountain. Lightweight is key! Also don't forget some waterproof trousers. There is nothing worse than feeling wet and miserable with 2 hours of walking to get back to your car. There's all the gear you need now it's time to get walking! Always bring a mobile phone with you and remember to bring some food and fluid.

Not only can you get fit with hill walking, but you can make new friends. There are hundreds of clubs across the country that walk at weekends and organise regular trips which provide a great way to meet new people. What more are you waiting for, now get out, get active and feel alive in this wonderful country of ours!

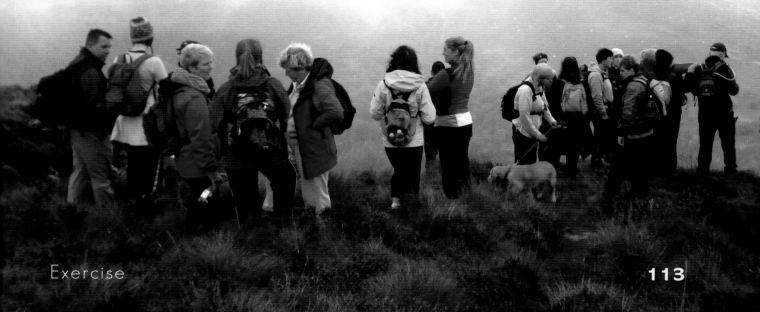

Computer-based fitness games

In the past few years, there has been a huge increase in the number of computer games that are being developed for the fitness market. In my opinion, this is a brilliant development because, just like this book, it brings fitness into your home, away from all the public fitness areas that people can feel so self-conscious in.

In short, the games do two things, simulate sports and get you to do exercises. The sports simulations can be fun and actually burn a surprising number of calories, the workouts will be somewhat effective, no question about it. I feel that these games are great for all the family too, as they can make fitness fun and can also be done indoors when the weather is bad.

Are they as good as the real thing? Possibly not, but they aren't too far off. I have been lucky enough to do some work with EA Sports and have to say that I am impressed with the development of their new fitness games such as ea sports active.

If you feel too self-conscious to work out, then this could the route for you. These games will help teach you the basics of fitness and will get you off the couch, which is always a good move.

Sex

This is possibly the most enjoyable form of exercise there is, I have always raved about its qualities.

Some years ago, celebrities such as Kelly Brook and Martine McCutcheon swore by sex as a way to stay fit and even released books about it. Sex is a great exercise tool and possibly one of the easiest ways to burn off those calories and have fun at the same time. Sex 3 times a week can cut the risk of a heart attack in half, according to a Queen's University study. The same 3 times per week will also burn an average 6 Big Macs annually.

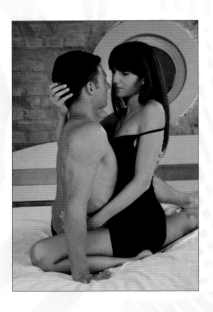

Let's call this sexercise. No, I am not messing with you, sex is a fantastic and enjoyable way of exercising! Just like gym training, sex will do the following:

▸ Increase your cardiovascular fitness.

▸ Improve your circulation.

▸ Increase blood flow in your body.

▸ Release endorphins, the happy hormones.

- Burn calories, roughly 400 per hour!

- Improve your strength.

Sex is a fab way of working certain muscles, such as your pelvis, arms, bum and your legs. But to really rev up your sex life, why not combine the two. By exercising, you can improve your sex life no end. When you train and get results you increase your self-esteem and your sex drive too. Giving yourself more confidence about your body, this, in turn, obviously helps when the lights go off …

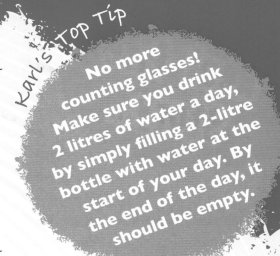

Karl's Top Tip

No more counting glasses! Make sure you drink 2 litres of water a day, by simply filling a 2-litre bottle with water at the start of your day. By the end of the day, it should be empty.

There are 3 areas that you can train to help further improve your sex life:

- **Your cardiovascular fitness:** You have no better excuse than this to get yourself up on to that cross trainer for 30 minutes.

- **Your flexibility:** Work on stretching out those hamstrings and quads, maybe a little yoga to help you on your way.

- **Your pelvic floor muscles:** Try this exercise. Lie on the ground, knees bent and hands by your side. Now kick your pelvis up in the air toward the ceiling and repeat 30 times.

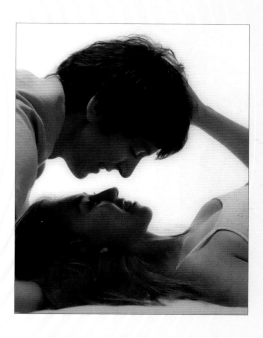

These 3 areas will give you great improvements in burning those calories away and with all the increase in exercise you will have even more energy. This then leaves you free to go home and exercise some more! Ha, but on a serious note it really is that good. Sex is nature's way of protecting the body too, by releasing beneficial hormones and chemicals such as:

- **Endorphins:** The happy hormone, helps to combat depression.

- **Cortisone:** Acts as an anti-inflammatory.

- **Oestrogen (in women):** Helps to combat osteoporosis.

- **Dopamine/norepinephrine:** Give a sense of euphoria.

- **Immunoglobulin:** Increases the effectiveness of the immune system.

Need I give you anymore reasons? By doing a little work in the gym, then hopefully a lot more at home, you can get in fantastic shape and feel amazing too. Who said that exercise couldn't be fun?

I am five feet ten inches tall, in my mid-fifties and would be a size fourteen.

Up to the age of forty, keeping fit never really interested me. I would go to the gym and basically do my own thing and that seemed to work up to a point. Then, I started to put on a bit of weight and my clothes size gradually crept up size fourteen – nothing much, but enough to bother me. So for my birthday, my partner gave me twelve gym sessions and so began my on/off love affair with keeping fit and exercise.

I loved what keeping fit did to my body but did not enjoy the process, so having someone point me in the right direction really worked for me. The keeping fit aspect of it was a by-product of the sessions, for me, it was all about losing the flabby bits.

This new-found fitness came in to its own in June 2009 when I slipped coming out of a friend's house and broke my ankle. I needed an operation and am now the proud owner of screws and plates in my ankle. Being somewhat fit helped, although I did not see it at the time and it was good to know that while my leg was in plaster, there were exercises that I could do that would help maintain some level of fitness so that when the plaster came off after six weeks, I did not feel that I had to go right back to the beginning.

After a couple of months, I could feel my energy and my fitness levels improving. Also, while in plaster, I was able to do leg raises which certainly helped when the cast came off. A year on from my accident, I find that regular exercise helps keep by ankle fairly supple.

I also find that exercise is a great trade off – if I behave myself during the week, do my cardio work and my gym work, eat sensibly (or as someone says 'keep your food tight') then, at the weekend, I can take a night off and indulge myself in whatever takes my fancy without the guilt. So for a little bit of hard work and self-discipline, I can have my nights out guilt free!

Over the years I have found that keeping fit is not only good for my body but also my mind, I feel energised after a long walk, even problems don't seem to be insurmountable after exercise.

So for a few hours effort a week, I have the satisfaction of knowing that I am keeping fit as I get older.

Exercising while pregnant

Despite what many people think, pregnancy doesn't mean that you have to stop training and put on a lot of weight – you simply need to modify your programme to suit your body. You can still achieve a great body and stay healthy while pregnant, keeping up all the gains that you have made over the previous months.

Maternal obesity is the single biggest predictor for childhood obesity, so it is up to you to get fit and keep fit for the sake of yourself and your baby. Normal weight gain for pregnancy is on average 35 pounds, so keep an eye on how much weight you are putting on.

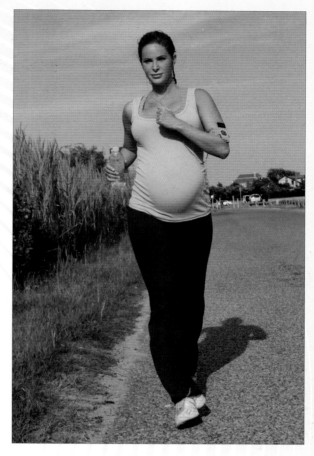

I have had several clients who took up exercise while pregnant and they did amazingly well, toning up and getting fit – and their bodies stayed toned and firm all the way through their pregnancies! James Clapp MD reported in 1996 that women who exercised during pregnancy had their babies an average of 5 days earlier than non-exercisers and had less need for medical intervention. In his paper to *The American Journal of Sports Medicine* he stated: 'The active phase of their labours is about 2 hours shorter, clinical and laboratory evidence of fetal stress is decreased, and the incidence of operative delivery (forceps or caesarean section) is reduced from 48 per cent to 14 per cent.'

Not only is it healthier for your baby, it is healthier for you too. Think, by doing just 30 minutes of exercise per day, you can have an easier and healthier pregnancy. This exercise doesn't even have to be gym work, as I will show you. The benefits of exercise during pregnancy is not just physical, due to your brain producing the endorphins that I am always talking about when you exercise, you are also less likely to have mood swings, pregnancy-specific stress and depression. However, the less active you are, the more emotionally unstable you are likely to be all the way through your pregnancy.

It is essential to be selective about the type of exercise you do when you're pregnant though. Obviously bouncing or jumping movements are out, as are running and aerobics (in the final trimester). Any movements that place excess stress on your lower back or pelvic area are also a definite no, no, but that leaves a whole world of exercise that is open to you.

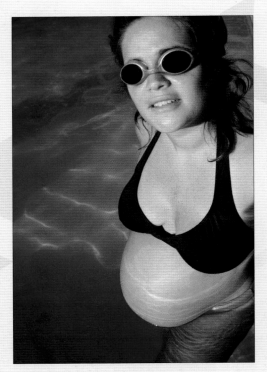

Swimming

Swimming is fantastic as it alleviates stress on your lower back and takes the pressure off your joints too. When you are in the water, there is less pressure on your body as a whole than there would be with other forms of exercise. Many pools have specific classes on for pre- and post-pregnancy women, so see if your local pool have any specific pregnancy classes on at the moment and why not try them, you might just enjoy it!

Yoga

The gentle movements of yoga are great for pregnant women and it's a fantastic way to relax for you too. Every yoga centre will have at least one class for pregnancy, it really is one of the easiest ways to exercise while you're pregnant, and provides you with a great social outlet too.

Exercises such as side leg raises and dumbbell work are great for toning the body and, when done correctly and gently, will actually increase your muscle tone all the way through your pregnancy. Keep the movements controlled and if you want to do the dumbbell exercises that I will show you later in this section, ensure that you are seated so that all the pressure is taken off your lower back.

Walking

In the early stages of pregnancy, walking is a great way of keeping fit.

When you do start training, don't over do it. Keep your heart rate down to around 140 beats per minute. The easiest way to do this is take the talk test. Always ensure that you are able to talk while you exercise, there will be less oxygen in your system available for exercise, so be careful not to push yourself too hard. Always breathe out when you are pushing against a force or weight and breathe in on the easy part of the exercise.

It is easy to decide to stop exercising when you are pregnant, but there is no proof to support the fact that this is necessary. As I have shown you, exercise will not only deliver great results physically for you, it will make your pregnancy easier, even making your labour easier. What's stopping you from exercising now?

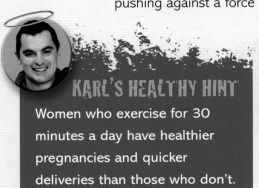

KARL'S HEALTHY HINT

Women who exercise for 30 minutes a day have healthier pregnancies and quicker deliveries than those who don't.

Eating for sport

If you are already quite active and want to improve your performance, one of the easiest ways to do this is by ensuring that you are eating properly. Over the years, I have learned the hard way just how important food can be. There are 3 important timeframes to analyse when you are training for sports.

▸ The pre-activity fuel.
▸ The during-activity fuel.
▸ The post-activity fuel.

The pre-activity fuel

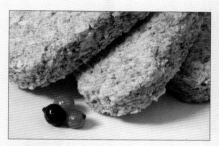
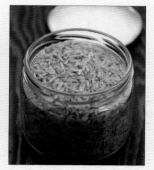

Ideally taken the night before as well as the morning of, this meal should be high in carbohydrates. This will help to top up your glycogen stores, ensuring that you have plenty of energy. Foods such as brown pasta, brown rice and sweet potatoes for dinner are fantastic, the morning meal should consist of a carbohydrate-based cereal, such as Weetabix or Bran Flakes and even some brown bread toast with some jam. The jam will give you a nice bit of energy in the form of sugar.

The during-activity fuel

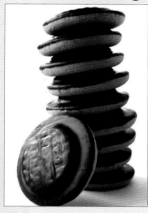

This does depend on the sport but, in general, you should be looking to eat and drink during the activity. For longer, endurance-based events that are over 2 or 3 hours, I would recommend eating every 30 minutes and sipping a drink every 15 minutes. This can vary from person to person, but all too often, people don't get enough food into their bodies.

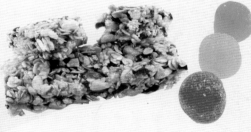

Foods that are ideal are Jaffa cakes, granola bars, chocolate bars and jellies. These are all high in sugar, giving your body plenty of energy that is readily available. In terms of fluid, I would recommend either water or a sports drink that has some simple sugars in it, such as Lucozade sport. For the very long endurance events, people will use high-sugar drinks such as Coke and 7Up. Be careful using these as the energy from these will last a short time, generally around 20 minutes or so, leading to a very fast drop in energy afterwards.

When racing a good friend from Clonakilty to Castlegregory on racing bikes, I was amazed to see that Coca-Cola was his fluid of choice, going through at least 6 litres over the course of 200 kilometres.

The post-activity fuel

This is the crucial part that many people forget about. Post-workout, your body needs to get nutrients within 30 minutes for the best recovery. If you fail to get the nutrients in, then you will be slower to recover, be stiffer, have worse muscular stiffness and less energy.

The easiest way to get all your nutrients in is in a drink form. You should aim to get a ration of 4:1 in terms of carbohydrate to protein for optimum recovery. Drinks such as Yazoo will do this perfectly, we even use a product called Ensure, which is a meal replacement drink for older people. By having this meal, you will be fresh and ready to go for your next session, yet it is the meal that most people forget about. Fruit will also help you here, citrus fruits being very effective but the drinks are so handy that you can just keep them in the back of the car and chances are you will use them more often.

What type of gym goer are you?

Are you a gym goer or do you prefer training at home? Take this quiz to find out.

▸ Do you stay motivated by yourself?

▸ Are your self-conscious when exercising in public?

▸ Do you get distracted easily?

▸ Do you find it hard to stick to definite workout times?

If the answer is yes to the above, then you are definitely better when working out at home.

▸ Do you love being around other people and enjoy meeting new people?

▸ Do you need the external motivation of classes?

▸ Do you like having lots of machines around you?

▸ Do you thrive off structure and having time put aside for working out?

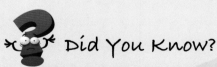 Did You Know?

If the answer is yes to these questions, then you would get great results from working out in a gym environment.

The human head weighs on average between 8 and 12 pounds, that's nearly 1 stone!

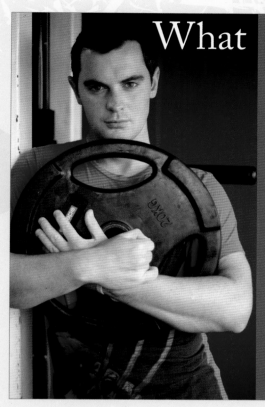

What happens when you work out with weights?

When you work out, you are placing stress on the muscle fibres in the area you are working. By placing minute tears on the muscle fibres, over time they grow back firmer and stronger, giving you muscle tone in that area. It's that simple.

Try this to demonstrate it for yourself. Extend your fingers wide and interlock them, this is your muscle before you train it. Now gradually pull the fingers apart, this is what happens when you train, the muscles get minute tears in them. Now bring the hands back together with your fingers together, this is your muscles fibres when then have been trained, they grow back firmer and stronger.

Setting up your home gym

More and more people are putting gyms into their homes, providing a convenient way to ensure that they get their workouts done. However, often these machines end up being nothing but glorified clothes horses, gathering dust and getting sold a few years later for a fraction of the price that was originally paid for them!

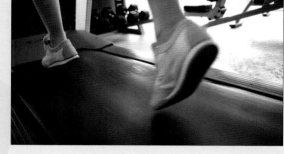

Here is my guide for you to ensure that your home gym doesn't end up just gathering dust. If you are going to spend the money putting a gym in, then let's make sure that you put the right type in. I have walked into the home gym of many of my new clients to see that they have bought machines that they didn't need, or will ever use. Home gyms don't need to be complicated – you don't even need that many machines! Let's take a look at exactly what you need to ensure that your home gym is exactly what you need.

First, you need to decide where you want to put your gym. There is no point buying too much equipment and cramming the room so that you have no space to work out! Or if you place the gym in a room that you don't like, you won't use it! For example, if you put a machine in an outhouse then when it's cold or it rains, you will decide to stay by

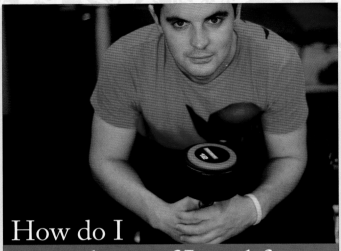

How do I know if I am lifting the right weight?

This is so, so easy to work out. You should be aiming to working hard towards the end of your reps. By this, I mean that on the last 2 reps of your exercise, you should be struggling a little. If you are aiming to do 20 reps, then 19 and 20 should be hard. If you are struggling on rep 10, then the weight is far too heavy and it should be lessened. Similarly, if you are doing 20 reps and you're not feeling anything at all, then it's far too easy, you need to make things slightly heavier.

Never ever buy equipment with out a warranty, because if it breaks, then you will have to spend more money to get it fixed. Providing another excuse for you not to use it!

When buying equipment, don't be afraid to try it before you buy it. This may sounds obvious but people often forget. Ask to have a full demonstration of what the machine can do and then try it for yourself. Some machines might be too small or too big to suit your body frame, so checking this is an essential part of buying a machine.

the fire. Choose a room that the equipment will fit in to, that you like using and that has a television. Chances are you will use the machine if you can watch a match or the news or your favourite programme.

The next thing you need to decide is who will be using it and what type of training they will be doing.

If you have knee problems, there is obviously no point in getting a treadmill! It is essential that you get equipment that suits your needs; great equipment is no use if you can not use it! If you have tried a machine in the gym and decided that you hated it, well I am afraid that things won't change if you get that machine for your house!

Ensure that you equipment comes with a full warranty, parts and frame, for at least 2 years. A warranty is your security in the event of there being a problem with the equipment, it is essential to have one.

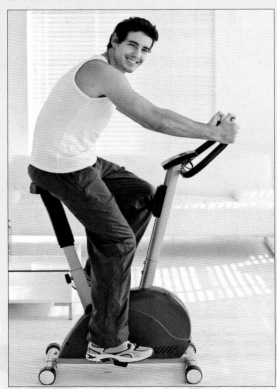

What machines should you buy?

You have a room, the motivation is there, so what machines should you buy? Some machines are essential for a home gym, obviously it is going to depend on your budget, but you will be surprised just how little you need.

Here are my recommendations

Cardiovascular

I recommend either a treadmill or a cross trainer as cardiovascular equipment. Treadmills can be great if you find it hard to walk or run outside, cross trainers are fantastic for people with knee or hip problems as the movement tends to be free flowing! However, it is essential to test these machines out, as different brands have different movements. In terms of treadmills, the important point is the level of absorption the belt has. The more absorption, the less pressure that will be placed on your joints, so, if you can, go for the more expensive option. Cheaper treadmills have less absorption and place more pressure on your joints, which is not good!

Resistance training

Depending on your budget, you have two options here. The first option is to get an adjustable bench and some dumbbells, which enable you to do a wide variety of exercises by simply changing the angle of the bench. For those of you on a tight budget, this would be my recommendation. Ensure you get a good range of dumbbells, as you get stronger you will need heavier weights.

If you have a bigger budget, I would highly recommend a multigym as well as the adjustable bench. A multigym is a machine that enables you to do a large variety of exercises, especially when combined with an adjustable bench. There are different types and sizes, just make sure that they will fit into your room!

Other equipment

The only other essential pieces of equipment that you need would be a soft mat, such as a yoga mat, and then you really are good to go!

All that you need to do now is to get into the gym and start working out! I have seen home gyms with numerous other extras such as plasma televisions with surround sound, swimming pools and hot tubs to name but a few accessories, while these are all fantastic, the pieces of equipment listed above are the essentials to establishing a great home gym.

How much will it cost me?

Home gyms can cost anything from €1,200 upwards. But don't be fooled by cheap equipment, ensure that you get a good warranty and that the company you buy from will provide you with good after-sales service. Cheap equipment simply won't last long, the warranties tend to be very poor and in terms of cardio equipment, cheap really is nasty! So try to avoid at all costs. You will be amazed at the deals that are being done at the moment, so go and bargain and get that gym that you always wanted!

Going to a gym

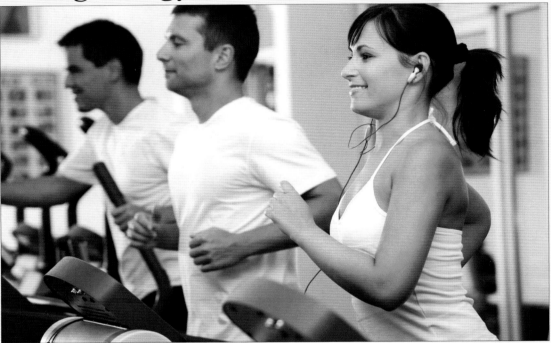

When you join a gym for the first time, it can be a really scary experience, if you look out for a few things, you'll soon feel at ease.

▶ Try to ensure that the gym is close to your home or your work place.

▶ Check it has all the facilities that you want. Do you want a pool or classes?

▶ When you are being shown around the gym floor are there any instructors around or is everyone left to their own devices? This is important as most gyms provide very little or no service unless you are paying extra, small gyms are better in this regards as they may not have the facilities but you can be sure that you will be given more service and have more interest taken in you than in the larger gyms.

The key factor is that you feel comfortable with the environment and the people you are dealing with, these are the people that are going to help you get fit so you need to trust them.

Gym etiquette

When you have joined, what is the etiquette for using the gym?

I am going to tell you about the dos and don'ts of going to the gym, how to avoid the cringe moments that we all hate so much. Having been around gyms for a long, long time, I have seen my fair share of these moments, while some of the points that I make may seem a little amusing, I guarantee that they are important to making your (and everyone else's) gym experience all the better.

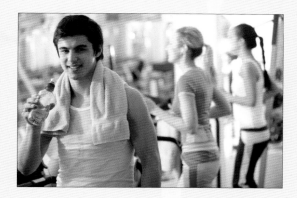

The definite gym no-nos:

▷ Sorry to have to break the news, but spandex is out! The ultimate cringe clothing should never be worn; it went out of fashion along with Mr Motivator in the early 1990s!

▷ Knee-length socks should also be left at home or kept for the soccer pitch.

▷ Never, ever, ever train in your bare feet. Most gyms have banned this as it is unhygienic for other gym users.

▷ If you are wearing runners, for everyone's sake, please ensure that they don't smell. Along with damp clothing, smelly runners can be nasty!

▷ Mirrors are there to make sure you are doing the exercise properly, not for posing in, so no mirror hogging.

▷ Here's one for the guys: don't try to injure yourself by using weights that are too heavy for you, and no screaming or yelling like a caveman please. Women aren't impressed by this, you may be sorry to hear.

▷ If you want to use your own music in the gym, don't try to burst your ear drums with the loudness; others may not want to listen to your music.

▷ Last but possibly most importantly, try to avoid training without using deodorant first! Especially for the guys as men have a tendency to suffer from smelly pores more than women. This can be very off putting!

Some important dos:

▷ Always take a towel with you in a gym and when you are finished on a machine, wipe it down so that the next person can use it. The last thing someone else wants is to lie on a bench covered in your sweat.

▷ Low-cut ankle socks are all the trend, so we are loving them. They can also make your legs look longer too which is always good.

▷ Always try to have some water with you, this will help you to keep hydrated while training.

▷ Fitted training clothing is always good too, but be careful that it's not too fitted. Try to wear clothing that you feel comfortable in, as you will always train better in clothing that you like.

▷ Guys, if there is a woman approaching and you are near a door, then have some manners and open the door for them. Men in the new affluent Ireland seem to have forgotten their basic manners. This also applies if you and a woman are waiting for a machine, why not let the woman go first? I am an old-fashioned guy and believe that men should have some old-school manners, even in the gym.

Training in a gym should be a great experience and one that is enjoyed by everyone. Just be careful that your enjoyment doesn't infringe on someone else's.

Exercise techniques on the market

I feel the workouts in this book will get you better results than the options listed below, and in the comfort of your own home too, but every bit of exercise helps.

▸ **Swiss balls:** Swiss balls are the big multicoloured balls that are in your local gym – though many of you may have them in your home. Swiss balls were originally used by elite athletes to improve balance/core strength during workouts and were then rolled (pardon the pun) out to the mainstream market. They can be great to use instead of a bench for certain exercises and do have some great benefits, but you won't find them in the exercises in this book, I feel that, unless supervised, they can be dangerous.

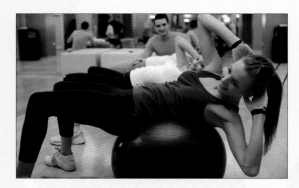

▸ **Power Plates:** Power Plates, or Vibroplates, have been in the market for the past 4 years or so and have seen a huge marketing/sales push in recent times. Basically, the idea is that you stand on a platform that vibrates. The more the plate vibrates the harder the exercise should become. Having tested one of the best models a few years back, I wasn't impressed. I feel that the idea of sending a vibration through your joints can damage the joints and have seen this occur twice. I certainly think that they may be useful for rehabilitation work but for getting fitness results, I fail to see the benefits.

▸ **Kettlebells:** Kettlebells have been around since the beginning of the weight-lifting scene and have made a resurgence recently. Basically, they are a kettle shaped dumbbell and, because of their shape, there are a range of different exercises that you can do with them. The workouts are tough and they can be a nice change from other classes. I do feel that some of the exercises performed with Kettlebells are far too advanced for the mainstream market, but many of the exercises are quite good.

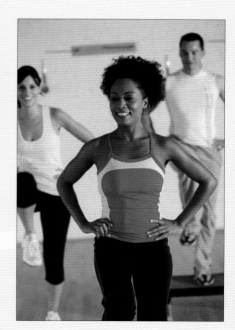

▸ **30-minute workouts:** Several years ago, the niche of 30-minute sessions hit Ireland and expanded rapidly throughout the country. They were cheap to set up and easy to market. All in all, they got people moving and that in my book is always a positive. I certainly feel that workouts need to be around an hour in duration to get the best results and the best workouts, but 30 minutes is better than nothing. Use these workouts as part of an overall plan with food and cardiovascular work and you will make good progress for sure as they will help.

Gym classes

Gym classes provide a structure to your training and access to a qualified professional. When looking for a class, you should get a good instructor who screens you before the class begins for injuries/medication, etc. Ideally try to get to a class that is small – the bigger the class, the less attention you will receive. By finding a good, small class, you will get more attention from the instructor and the chances are that you will be doing the exercises with better technique.

Another element that I feel is very important is the shape of the instructor taking the class. They have probably been teaching the class for some time and their body has adapted to that. By looking at the body of the instructor, you will be able to see what muscles are developed by doing that class. This is only used as a very rough guide but sometimes can be quite accurate.

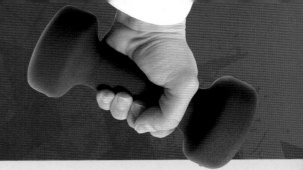

There are so many different types of class on the market and all do slightly different things. If you are a little confused by what they all mean, here is a quick guide to some classes that may be on in your local area.

Spinning

Spinning is an exercise class that simulates a cycling experience on a stationary bike in a class setting. It was created by Jonathan Goldberg in 1987 in the USA. No gym or instructor is allowed to use the term spinning unless they are authorised by Goldberg's company.

The instructor will lead the class on his/her bike and will have loud music in the background – spinning is a tough class. Using music and microphones, you will be pushed to do your best. The instructor will vary the class by varying positions, etc.

The effort level is changed in three main ways:

▸ by varying the resistance on the flywheel;

▸ cadence-by pedalling faster/slower;

▸ by sitting or standing in different positions.

You will generally have a heart monitor during the class to see what your heart rate is and what training zone you are in.

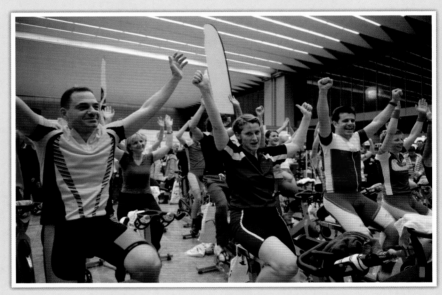

So what's the problem? Some trainers, myself included, think that if you do too much spinning, your calves and legs can actually get bigger. Next time you see a cyclist on the road, have a look at their calves, most of the time they will be chunky. Big calves on women will make their legs look shorter and stumpier, and very few women I know want that. Now I don't mean that by doing 1 class a week or every 2 weeks you will get bigger calves, but I do think that doing too many spinning classes in a week can do this to you. Yes you will be burning a lot of calories, getting fitter and reducing stress, but you should vary your exercise.

Spinning if used properly and not too often is a good thing, but if it is overdone, or not done properly, it is dangerous. Problems such as back and knee injuries are associated with overdoing spinning as well as the gains in leg size that I mentioned earlier. The other important element to remember is that you drink lots of water during your session.

Real Results

Boot camp

In recent years, boot-camp classes have taken over the country, and are mostly run in parks and beaches. Boot camps include exercises from all different types of class and also add in plenty of cardiovascular workouts too, for an all-over workout. Tough, social, outdoors and easy on the pocket, these classes provide a gruelling workout that targets every different component of fitness.

It is important that you give a full medical screening to your instructor before you begin and it is also important that you have a group which is relatively small in size. The smaller the group, the more attention that you will get from the instructor. Because of the type of classes there is an increased risk to injuries etc., especially in the winter when the ground is soft and mucky.

Circuit

Circuit classes are a little bit different to body sculpting. There will be several different stations or exercises and you simply rotate in a circuit and do each exercise before moving on to the next.

There can be a few different types of circuit and you either have to do a certain number of repetitions or spend a certain amount of time before moving on to the next station. This type of class provides a great workout for all your muscle groups and, because of the nature of the circuit, you get lots of attention from the instructor which is always good!

Did You Know?

Sit-ups won't give you a flatter stomach. We all have six-packs, it is what covers them that differentiates us. It is estimated that you would need to do 250,000 sit-ups to burn 1 lb of fat from your body!

Body sculpting

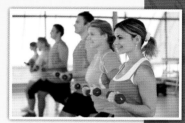

Body-sculpting classes are group-based classes that are developed to tone and sculpt the muscles using variations and combinations of exercises using your body weight and light dumbbells. These classes can be a great way to sculpt your body, normally the reps are quite high and the instructor will be at the top of the class.

Again, it is essential that you get a good instructor to teacher your class. The instructor should screen you for injuries, etc. and also give you attention during the class to correct you if you are doing something the wrong way. This is one of the key factors that I think all instructors should adhere to and very many don't. Not everyone in a class scenario will be able to follow every exercise and the instructor should give you as much attention as possible.

Bums and Tums

Normally a shorter class of 20 or 30 minutes, this is a great way to get lots of exercises for the stomach and bum with a qualified instructor. These classes can be easily fitted into your lunch break and will make a difference when the time comes to get into your bikini.

Interval training

Do you want to do less exercise and burn more calories? Not seeing results from spending hours on the treadmill? Then interval training is for you! Interval training makes your body work harder while you're exercising, increasing your heart rate and burning more calories.

It uses your body's two energy-producing systems: the *aerobic* and the *anaerobic*.

The *aerobic* system enables you to walk or run for several miles. It uses oxygen to convert carbohydrates from various sources throughout your body into energy that can be used for a long period of time.

The *anaerobic system* draws energy from carbohydrates (in the form of glycogen) stored in the muscles for short bursts of activity such as sprinting, jumping or lifting heavy objects. This system doesn't need oxygen, and can only last for several seconds. Its by-product, lactic acid, is responsible for that achy, burning sensation in your muscles that you feel after running up several flights of stairs.

Interval training enables you to enjoy the benefits of anaerobic activities without having to endure those burning muscles. A great trick is to tell yourself that you'll run a particular distance – for example, from the blue car to the green house on the corner – and then walk from the green house to the next telephone pole.

There are four ways to vary your interval training, simply pick one that suits you and you can get started.

- Speed.
- Time.
- Rest time.
- Reps.

Now that you have chosen what variable you want to use, the next element is to put your interval programme together. Simply make one variable easy and the second one hard. Ideally, look to get 1 hour in total from your workout. For example, if time is the variable that you are using, walk for 1 minute and then run for 1 minute.

See the table below for more examples in a very basic form.

Variable	Easy	Hard
Speed	6 kmh for 1 minute	10 kmh for 1 minute
Time	10 minutes walking	10 minutes jogging
Rest	1 minute rest every 10 minutes	30 seconds rest every 10 minutes
Reps	4 reps in total	10 reps in total

Interval training delivers the best benefits from minimal training. It is one of the best workouts for burning fat and can be done on any machine in your gym or out on the road. So what are you waiting for?

Real Results

There is a very simple method to help you recover safely and quickly, it is called the **RICE** technique.

Rest: If you feel a strain, stop exercising straight away. You need to rest up and let the muscle recover.

Ice: Apply ice to the injured area as this will help prevent (or will reduce) swelling. Swelling causes more pain and can dramatically slow down the healing process. Apply a cloth-covered ice pack to the injured area for no more than 20 minutes at a time, 4 to 8 times a day – applying ice more for than 20 minutes may cause cold injury or skin burn. Areas with little fat and muscle, such as fingers or toes, should only have ice on them for about 10 minutes. A 1-pound pack of frozen corn or peas makes a good ice pack. It is lightweight, conforms to the injured area, and is inexpensive and reusable. When making an ice pack with a plastic bag, make sure that all the air is out of the bag before closing it. Frozen gel packs are colder than ice, so they should only be left on for 10 minutes. Always check the skin every 5 minutes for and redness or swelling, if this occurs then take the ice off the skin.

Compression: Apply some strapping to the area or use a support, which can be bought from local sports shops. This helps to reduce the swelling in the area. Be careful not to bandage the area too tightly – if it throbs or hurts, then the bandage is on too tight.

Elevation: Elevation means raising the injured area above the level of the heart, which may involve lying down to raise a leg high enough. To help reduce swelling, the affected part should be elevated so it is 12 inches above the heart. Prop up a leg or arm while resting it, this can be done using several pillows.

This is the best way to treat an injury or strain initially. If the pain continues, then make an appointment with your GP or physiotherapist. It is also important to note that anyone with Raynaud's, diabetes, sensitivity to cold or any medical condition with reduced blood flow to the arms or legs should *not* use RICE therapy.

Know your muscle groups

Front

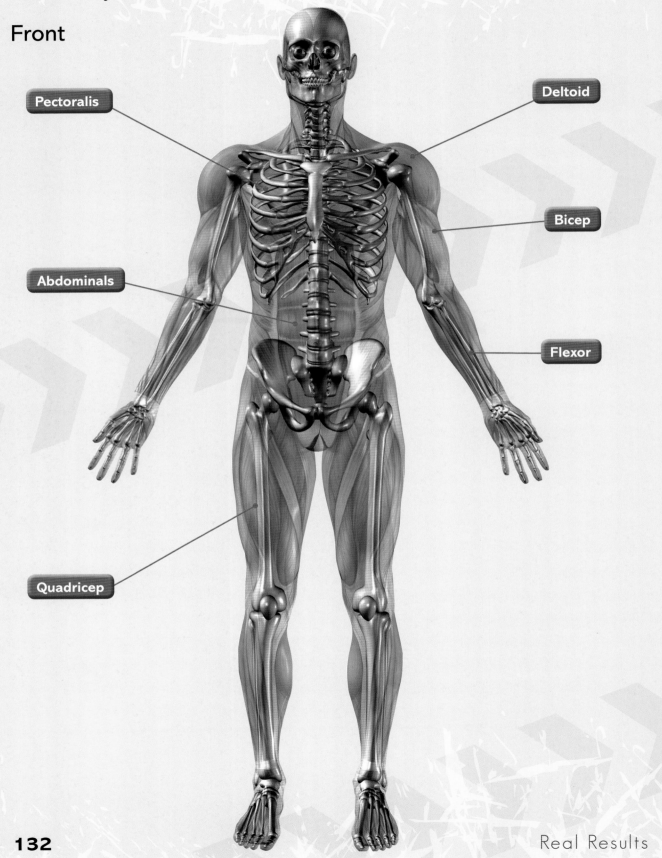

Pectoralis

Deltoid

Bicep

Abdominals

Flexor

Quadricep

Real Results

Back

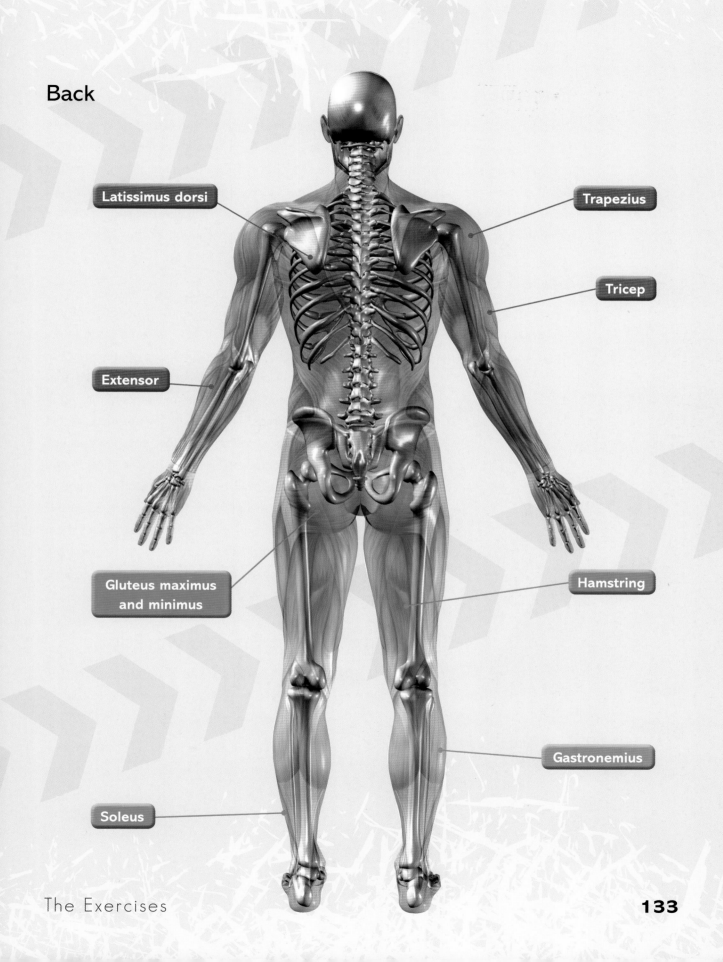

Latissimus dorsi

Trapezius

Tricep

Extensor

Gluteus maximus and minimus

Hamstring

Gastronemius

Soleus

Before you begin the workouts

Breathing

Not only will breathing keep you from fainting during exercise, new research also suggests that it may even help you lose weight. Many of us don't breathe properly – or at all – during exercise but you should always breathe out on the hard part of the exercise and breathe in on the easy part – it's as easy as that! By breathing properly, you will get more oxygen into your body, helping you to work out harder. You also reduce the chance of fainting or feeling sick during training as you are getting enough air into your body.

Speed of movements

This is one of the most important areas of any exercise programme. Speed is not just important in relation working the proper muscle groups, it also ensures your safety when you train, reducing the chance of injury. I always recommend that you go at

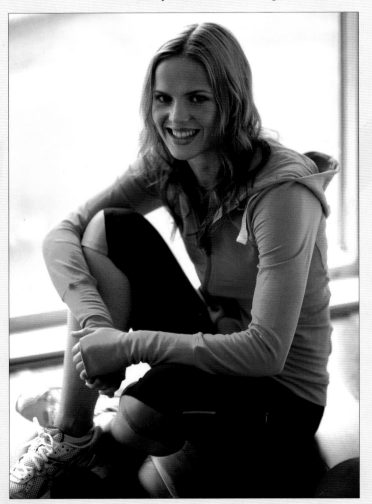

a controlled pace, not going too fast that you compromise the movement, making it dangerous. The form of the exercise should always come first, as this ensures that you are working the correct muscle groups and that the muscles are being worked properly. Often towards the end of a set, people will rush through the exercises just to get them over with, using every body part except the one they are meant to be working. So control, control, control!

Best time to workout

There are many answers to this question. The main answer is that the best time to train is the time that suits you best!

I personally don't like training in the morning, it just doesn't seem to suit me at all, so I get most of my training done in the evening. But if you love training in the morning, then that's the best time to train for you – and the same with evenings or afternoons.

Real Results

From a physical perspective, the morning tends to be the best time to train as you will then increase your metabolic rate for the whole day, burning more calories naturally! Sometimes, if you train late in the evening you may find it hard to sleep as you have endorphins rushing around your body, giving you that post-exercise adrenaline rush. So you will know yourself what time suits you to train the best. However, no matter what science says, if you don't like something, it is very hard to change that habit, so stick to what you like and you will help to make changes that will last for life.

The equipment needed

To do the workouts in this book, all you will need are a mat and 2 bottles of water (or 2 dumbbells). It really is that easy, no complicated Swiss balls or anything like that – remember we are looking to get you real results from real exercise! The more complications there are, the harder it will be for you to keep it up for a long period of time. These exercises can be done at home or in your gym, which ever suits you.

Stretching

Stretching is a controversial topic at the moment. In my opinion, it is essential to stretch at the end of the workout to loosen out the muscle fibres in the body parts that you have just worked on. Stretching at the beginning of a workout will do you no harm whatsoever, as long as you're not stretching too far. Remember at the beginning of a workout, your muscles are cold, and stretching too far on cold muscles may produce a strain or a tear, which is not good.

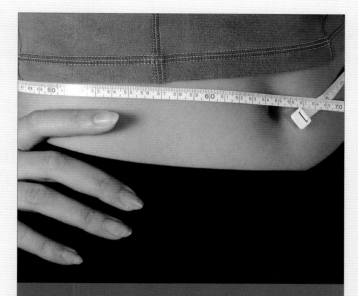

Core, core and more core

Core is one of the most overused words in the fitness industry. The 1990s and 2000s brought many things to the industry, an obsession with strengthening the 'core' was one of them.

Here is the first point to note: nearly all exercises that you do involve your core. Your core in the centre of your body, from your neck to your hips both front and back. While it is true that some people have an inherent weakness there and need to strengthen it, most of us will get all the strengthening we need from doing exercises such as squats, bench presses and nearly all other exercises. If you are an Olympic athlete or professional sports star, then an in-depth analysis and specific training may need to be done, but most of the population who are training do not need to be doing so much work for the 'core'.

Try this, simply aim to pull your belly button to your spine when doing any exercise to engage these muscles and get them working nicely.

Yoga corpsing

Yoga corpsing for the ultimate and simplest de-stressing tool there is.

Picture the scene, your having the busiest day of the year, you are stressed, seriously stressed. You wish there was something that in ten minutes would relieve that stress so that you can deal with the rest of your day. Guess what? There is.

Go into a quiet room and close the door. Ideally, this exercise should be done lying down on the floor but you can also do it sitting in your chair.

▷ Sitting or lying, close your eyes and turn your palms towards the ceiling.

▷ Focus on your breathing, taking a deep breath in and slowly exhaling, emptying your lungs of all the air.

▷ Repeat 6 times.

▷ Next, take a deep breath in and hold the air in your lungs for 15 seconds.

▷ Slowly exhale and feel the stress leaving your body as you do.

▷ Repeat 6 times.

▷ Breathe in and hold the air. I now want you to tense your calves as hard as possible and hold for 15 seconds.

▷ Breathe out and relax the calves as you do so. Repeat twice and then go through your body in the following order.
  – Legs.
  – Chest.
  – Arms.

▷ Next go back to focus on your breathing – take a deep breath in and then a deep breath out – and open your eyes when you feel ready.

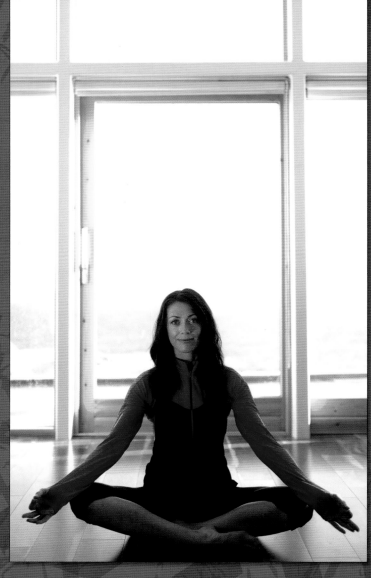

You will be amazed at just how chilled out you feel at the end of this simple sequence, you will be de-stressed and ready to tackle any obstacle that gets thrown at you, believe me.

I tend to recommend that people warm up using cardiovascular equipment in a gym or by doing light versions of the exercises first, if you feel the need to stretch after this, then you should. Stretching after a workout helps to relieve the post-exercise soreness that you may get a day or two after a workout.

So after completing your workout – be it my exercises in this book, your own session in a gym or on a surfboard or bike – here are some easy stretches that you can do to alleviate the pain.

Always hold a stretch for 15 to 20 seconds and do 2 sets. If you feel the need to do more, then do. I will show you one beginners' stretch for a body part and then a harder stretch to progress to.

You should never feel a lot of pain when you are stretching – if you are, it means that you are pushing yourself too far. A gentle stretch is nice, but a lot of pain more than likely means that you are doing some damage, so ease off. See how you go.

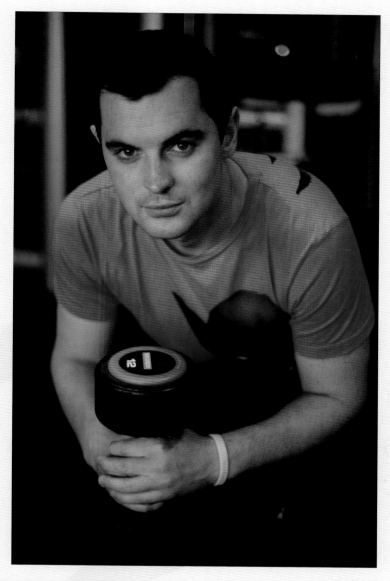

Body part	Easy stretch	Harder stretch
Front of leg	Quad stretch	Angled quad stretch
Back of leg	Standing hamstring stretch	Floor hamstring stretch
Arms	Tricep stretch behind neck	Hand pull in front
Back/shoulders	Door stretch	Assisted shoulder stretch
Neck	Side-to-side stretch	Hand assisted side to side
Lower back	The cat	The cobra

The Exercises

Front of Leg

Quad stretch

1. Stand facing a wall (for balance) with your feet together.

2. Take your right foot with your hand and bring it towards your bum. The important thing here is to ensure that the knees stay together. The more your knees separate, the less the quadriceps actually get stretched.

3. Change legs and repeat.

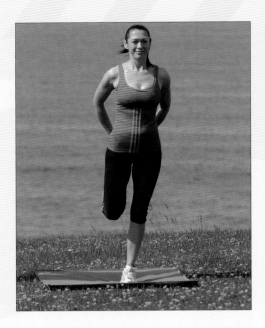

Angled quad stretch

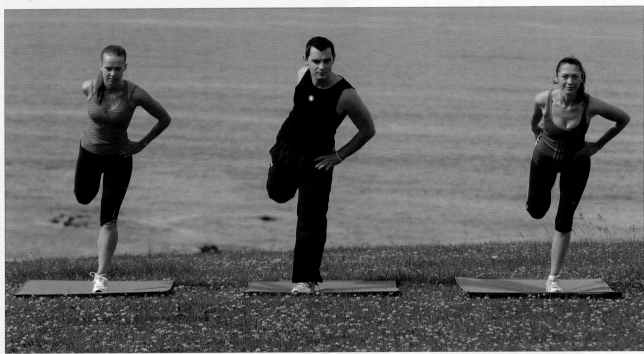

1. Stand facing a wall (for balance) with your feet together.

2. Take your right foot with your hand and bring it towards your bum. The important thing here is to ensure that your knees stay together. The more your knees separate the less the quadriceps actually get stretched.

3. While keeping the heel close to your bum, pull your leg back away from your body slightly. The farther the leg is pulled away, the more the stretch.

4. Change legs and repeat.

Real Results

Back of Leg

Standing hamstring stretch

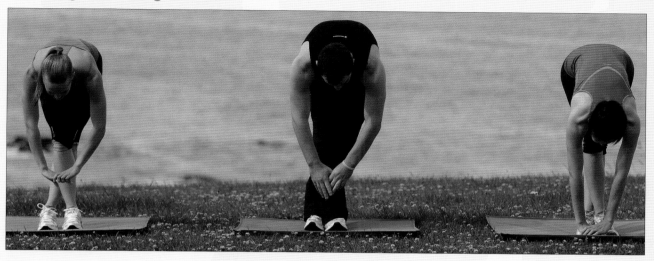

1. Stand with your feet together and your posture straight.
2. Cross your right leg over you left.
3. Gently bend down to reach your toes. If you find that you can't reach your toes, then just go as far as possible. The essential point is that you never bounce, always keep a controlled motion all the way through the stretch. Hold for 20 seconds.
4. Change legs and repeat.

Floor hamstring stretch

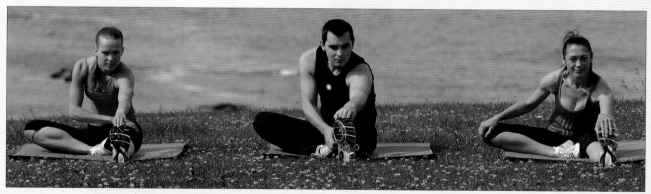

1. Start by sitting on the floor, with both your feet out in front of your body, bring your right leg to your left knee. Before you start, ensure that you are sitting tall, with a straight posture.
2. Simply bend forward and try to touch your toes, get as close as you feel comfortable. If you find this too easy, then simply try to get your elbows and forehead to your knees. As well as stretching your hamstrings this is also a great stretch for your lower back.
3. Change legs and repeat movement.

Arms

Tricep stretch behind neck

An easy and effective way to stretch out your arms, this one is mainly for the back of the arms.

1. Start with your right hand up in the air and your left hand at the base of your back.

2. Try to get your two hands touching behind your back. If you can't get them to touch then get a towel to place in between your hands, as you become more flexible then slide your hands down the towel until eventually they can touch.

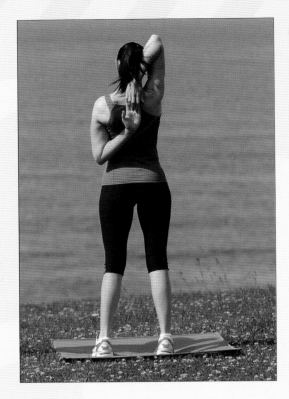

Hand pull in front

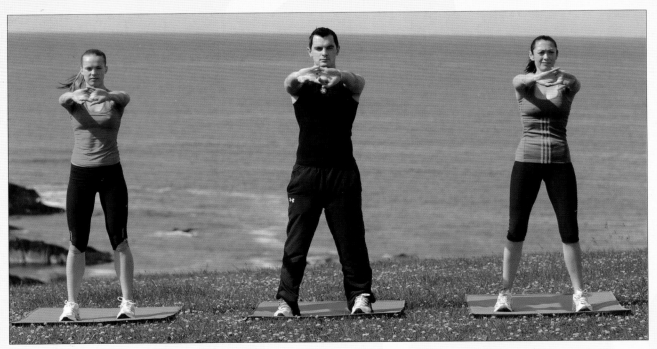

This stretch is a great way to stretch out the forearms and biceps.

1. Place your hands out in front of you, interlocking your fingers.

2. Extend your arms and gently push your palms away from you, keeping your arms extended. It may feel a little weird at first but over time you will grow to love this stretch.

Real Results

Back and shoulders

Door stretch

Another easy stretch, using simply the frame of your door.

1. Stand side on to the doorframe, resting your forearm against the frame.

2. Step forward and increase the stretch. The more you step forward the more of a stretch you will feel.

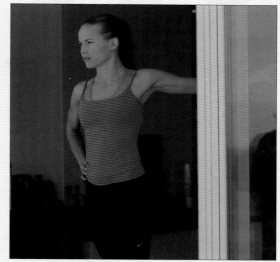

Assisted shoulder stretch

This stretch must be done with great care! While it is unbelievably effective, if overstretched you may damage your shoulders and we don't want that.

1. Sit at the end of the bench/bed with your stretching partner behind you.

2. Place your arms straight out to the side.

3. Your partner places their hands near yours and pulls your arms behind you. If they need more leverage they can place a foot midway up your back. You should be feeling a gentle stretch but nothing more than that, if you are then your stretching too far.

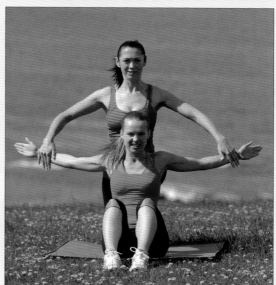

Neck

Side-to-side stretch

This is a great and easy to loosen out creaks and tightness in your neck.

1. Stand or sit straight and look forward, simply lean your neck to the left and hold it there. It's important to actually lean the neck to the side, not halfway between the side and the front.

2. Bring your head back to look forward and lean your neck to the right and hold it there.

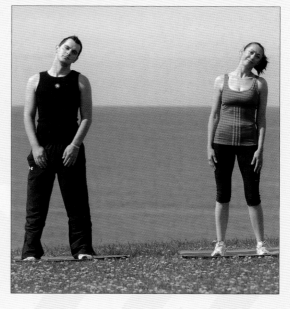

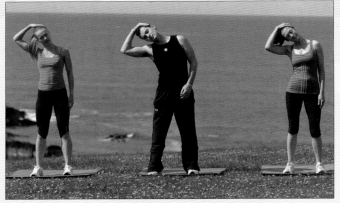

Hand assisted side-to-side

This is similar as the stretch above, except that you are using your hand to place pressure on the stretch. Be careful not to place too much pressure, just apply it gradually until you feel that you have enough.

Lower back

Cat pose

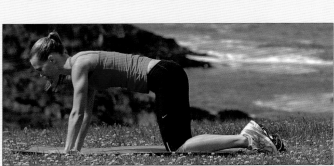

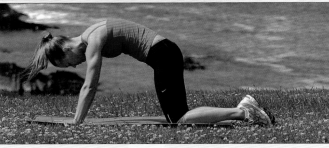

This is a yoga-based stretch that will loosen out even the stiffest of backs.

1. Get down on your mat on your hands and knees.

2. Push your spine towards the floor, gently, letting your stomach move to the floor.

3. Curl your back up towards the ceiling just like a cat would, pulling your belly button in towards your spine as you do. Breathe in on the up and breathe out on the way down.

Cobra pose

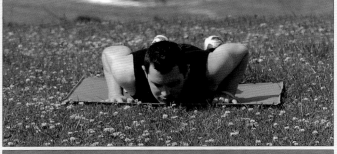

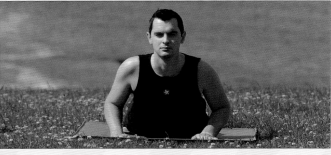

Another yoga posture and another great way to loosen out your spine.

1. Lie down on your mat on your stomach, with your hands placed by your shoulders, palms on the mat.

2. Keeping your belly button the mat, gently raise your upper body off the mat, using your hands for support. You should be moving 4 or 5 inches and not a whole lot more. There are variations of this stretch where you come farther up but, generally, I prefer this method.

The workouts

These workouts are designed for all levels of fitness, from the total beginner to the regular gym goer. They can be done in the comfort of your own home or in your local gym and require the bare minimum of equipment.

I have broken down each of the programmes, into body parts and there are two exercises per body part. This ensures that every one of your body parts gets worked properly and nothing is left out!

Everyone will have exercises that they love and exercises that they hate, but don't skip body parts, just knuckle down and get through it and, before you know it, you will have finished them.

Unless stated otherwise, you should aim to do 20 reps per exercise, beginning with 1 set and building up to 3 sets as your body gets stronger and stronger.

A **rep** equals the number of times you do the exercise in a set. For example, if you are doing sit-ups and want to do 3 sets of 20 reps, every sit-up is 1 rep and 20 sit-ups makes 1 set.

Remember that the goal for the workouts is not to have you so sore that you can't walk for a week after the session. All this will do is create a negative environment for you as you won't want to do the workouts again. A little pain is OK and to be expected, but too much pain is not good for anyone!

Warm up your body with the first few exercises and if you feel the need to stretch, then get a good stretch done and always stretch at the end of the workout to prevent stiffness, I know that sometimes it's the last thing you feel like doing but it will make a big difference to your body.

It's so important with all the exercises to follow good technique, with good posture. As your body fatigues, the first thing to change is generally your posture as it makes it easier for many of the movements. So chin up and chest out, straighten that back! The first time you do an exercise take it easy and get the movement right, then your can increase your pace of needs be from there.

9 Reasons to do weight training

Builds bone density
Increases strength
Helps firm up your body
Speeds up your metabolism
Helps to smooth and reduce cellulite
Improves your posture
Decrease dress size
Increases energy
Reduces stress

Beginners

This programme is designed for those of you who haven't exercised for a long time and who are just beginning your journey to get fit. The exercises will provide the building blocks for the harder exercises that will follow.

Because you are a beginner, you will see very rapid results, it's essential to make sure that you focus on the technique of the exercises and getting the basics right.

For week 1, just do 1 set of 20 reps 3 times in the week. In week 2, progress to 2 sets, 3 times a week and in week 3 do 3 sets 3 times a week. This ensures that you are easing your body into exercise and not doing too much too soon. As we saw earlier, doing too much too soon will leave you in a lot of pain and that is not the idea. There is no real need for you to be hurting badly after a workout, a little pain is good but not too much.

Let's take a look at the exercises.

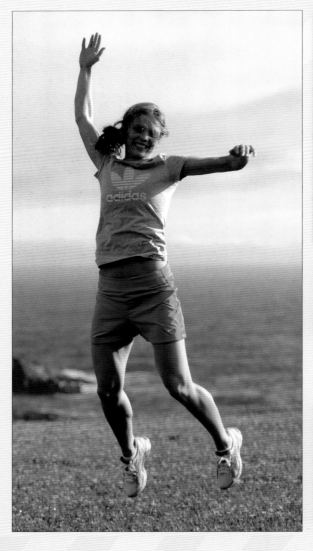

Bodypart	Exercise 1	Exercise 2
Legs	Squat	Lunge
Chest	Pec deck	Bench press
Back	Single-arm row	Bent-over row
Shoulders	Military press	Side lateral raise
Arms	Tricep dip	Bicep curl
Stomach	Regular sit-up	Bridge
Hips	Side leg raise	Bum kick

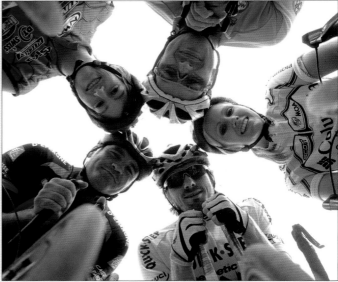

Real Results

Glossary

Squat   One of the oldest exercises in the book.

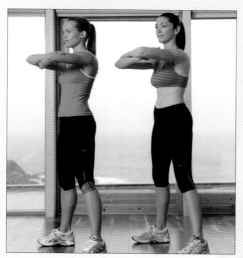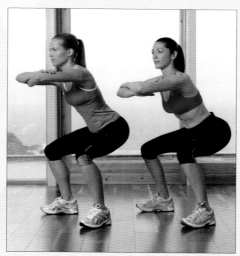

1. Stand with your feet shoulder-width apart.
2. Cross your hands at the front to keep your back straight.
3. Bend your knees as low as you feel comfortable. Many guidelines say 90 degrees, but not everyone is the same. Go as low as feels comfortable for you.
4. Return to the top.

Lunge

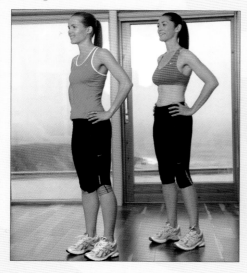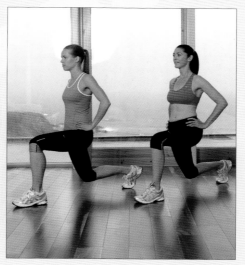

1. Stand with your feet together, your posture straight.
2. Lunge forward with your right leg, bending your left knee towards the floor. The important point to note is that the knee of the leading leg should never go over your foot. If this happens then simply take a bigger step forward.
3. Return to an upright position.
4. Repeat with your left leg.

Pec deck

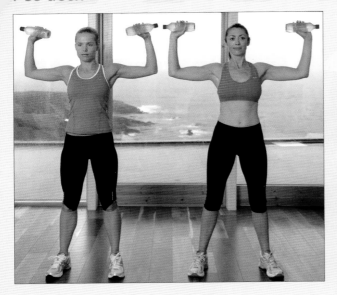 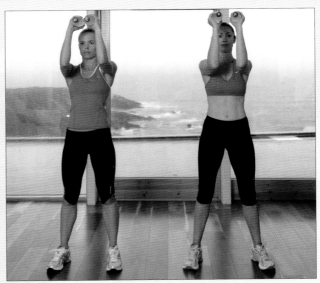

1. Stand with your feet shoulder-width apart.

2. Raise your elbows in front of you to 90 degrees in line with your shoulders.

3. Bring your elbows together. Try to make them touch in front of your body.
   If you begin to get neck pain then don't bring the elbows as close together.

4. Lower your elbows.

Bench press

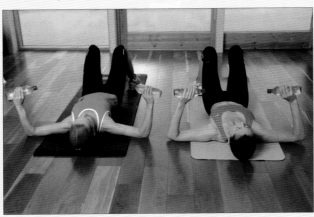 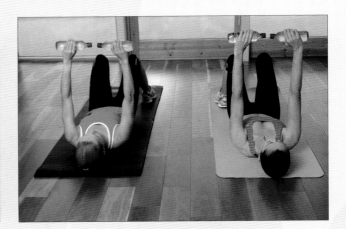

1. Lie on your back on your mat with your knees bent.

2. With a weight in either hand, extend your arms directly above your nipple line.

3. Lower your elbows to the floor in line with your shoulders.

Single arm row

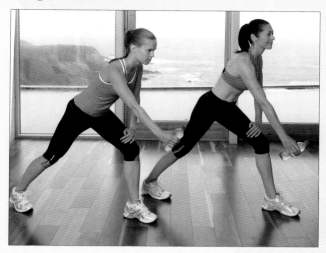 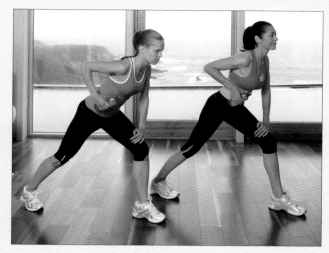

This is a fantastic back exercise.

1. Place one knee on a chair or bench or bend as above. Ensure that the other leg is straight and doesn't move during the exercise.

2. Place your hand on the chair to aid balance and ensure that your back is totally straight.

3. Extend your right arm to the floor and raise your left arm as high as you feel comfortable, keeping your elbow close by your body. Make sure that you extend your arm fully on the way down.

4. Return to an upright position.

5. Extending your left arm to the floor and raising your right arm.

6. Return to an upright position.

Bent-over row

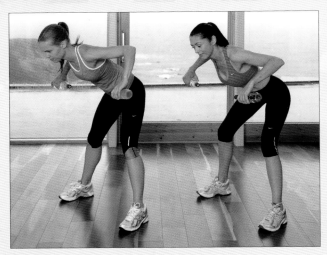 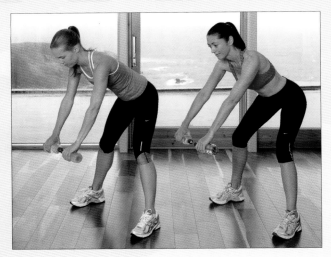

1. Stand with your feet wide apart.

2. Bend your knees as if you were sitting into a chair and tilt your upper body forward keeping your back straight.

3. Extend your arms fully towards the floor, keeping your hands with your palms facing your body and pull them up towards your body so that your elbows are higher or in line with your shoulders. Ensure that your arms are extended fully towards the floor.

4. Return to an upright position.

Military press

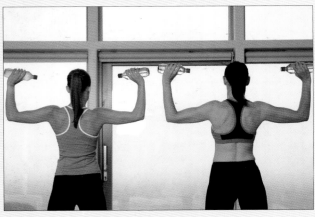 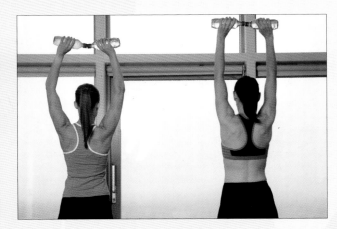

This is a totally old-school exercise.

1. Place your feet are shoulder-width apart for balance.

2. Holding the weights at each shoulder, push them straight towards the ceiling, touching in the middle.

3. Return the weights to your shoulders. Make sure that you bring them all the way down so that the weights touch your shoulders.

Real Results

Side lateral raise

This is a fantastic exercise for your shoulders.

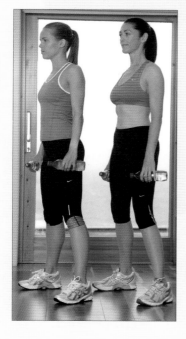 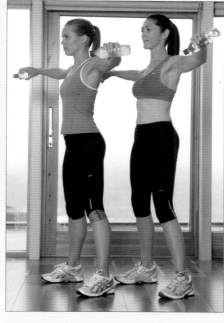

1. Place your feet shoulder-width apart.

2. Hold the weights by your hips, not in front of you. The important point with this exercise is that you pull your shoulders right back – don't let your shoulders round at the front when doing the exercise.

3. Raise the weights to the side, with a slight bend in your arms. Imagine you are pouring out water – as the weights rise, pour out the water. This engages the shoulders and gives you great definition.

4. Lower the weights back to your hips.

Tricep dip

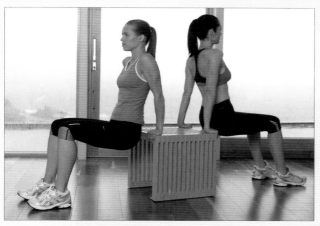 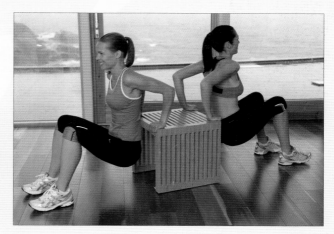

Time to hit those bingo wings.

1. Sit on a chair or bench.

2. Place your hands by your hips and your feet out in front, hamstrings parallel to the floor.

3. Bend your elbows so that your bum goes towards the floor. Always keep your bum close to the chair/bench, don't let it move away from it.

4. Extend your arms so that they are fully locked out. When you have completed all the reps, sit back on the chair.

To make this exercise harder, simply move your feet farther away from you.

Bicep curl

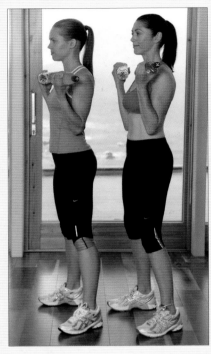 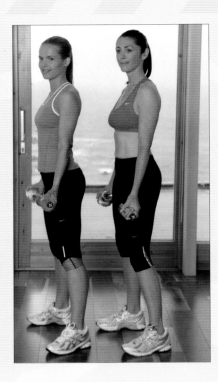

1. Stand with your feet shoulder-width apart, arms fully extended towards the floor, holding a weight in each hand.

2. Curl the weights up towards your shoulders.

3. Return to the starting position.

The important thing here is to keep your elbows close by your side, don't let them move away from the body as this means you aren't getting the most from your exercise.

Regular sit-up

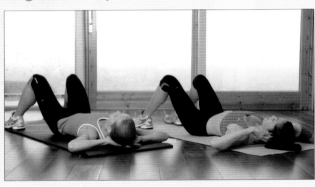 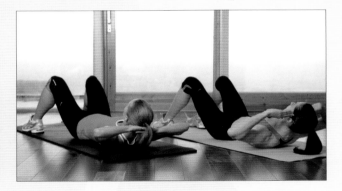

This is an old-school exercise that is generally done totally wrong. Here's the low down.

1. Lie on your back with your knees bent. The straighter your legs are, the more your lower back has to work.

2. Place your hands behind your head and ensure that your head is just resting in your hands, never pull your neck forward.

3. Pick a point on your ceiling and keep your eyes looking at that point all the way through.

4. Sit up about 3–4 inches, using your stomach, not your neck, and return to the floor.

If you have any neck pain, stop straight away. If you feel you are using your back, then place your feet up on a chair, to alleviate any pressure on your lower back.

Real Results

Bridge

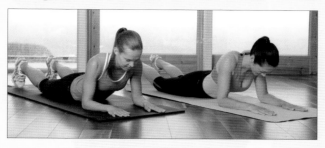 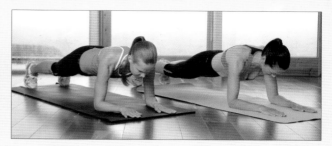

This exercise, more than most, will work your core.

1. Lie down on the mat on your stomach and place your elbows on the mat, just under your chest.

2. Keeping your knees at 45 degrees, raise your stomach off the mat keeping your back parallel to the floor.

3. Suck your belly button towards your spine and hold for 30 seconds initially – increase to 1 minute as you get stronger.

When this is easy, you can progress to the full bridge where your legs are totally off the floor, again ensuring that there is no dip in your back whatsoever. If you have any back pain at all then stop straight away.

Side leg raise

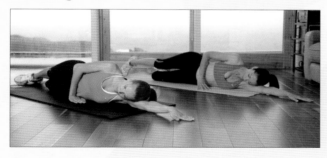 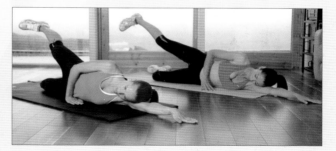

One of my favourite exercises for toning up the bum and hip areas.

1. Lie on your left side on the mat, ensuring all your joints are in one line. Your shoulders, hips, knees and ankles should all be in a straight line.

2. Point your toes towards your face and roll your hip to the front. This is the important trick, as it engages your hips/bum to work harder.

3. Raise your right leg as far as your feel comfortable and return your leg back to the starting position.

4. Repeat for your right side.

Watch that hip, always keep it rolled slightly frontwards!

Bum kick

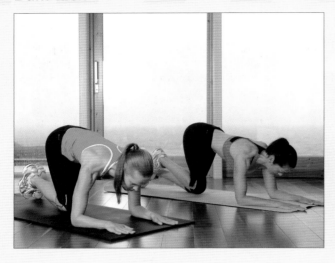 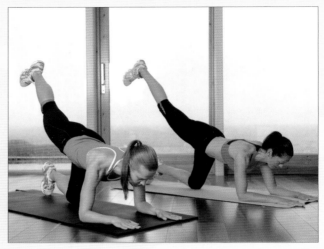

This is another old-school, Jane Fonda classic.

1. Get onto your mat, on all fours. Ensure that your shoulders and knees are body-distant apart.

2. Bring your right knee into your chest and then extend your leg fully back behind you. Make sure to kick your leg is higher than your bum. Ensure that your hips remain square all the time and that your back is flat.

3. Return to the starting position.

4. Repeat the exercise using your left leg.

If you find that you have any back pain then, obviously stop straight away.

Medium

You have now conquered the beginners' programme – your clothes are looser, your muscles more toned and you're feeling good about yourself. You're ready for the next challenge to keep those great results going.

As we discussed earlier, change is key to continuing to get great results, so with that in mind here is the next workout. It is more difficult, with new movements and exercises that will make you work harder and adapt quickly so you see results fast.

As always, exercise 3 times a week. Begin with 1 set of 20 reps and build up to 3 sets over the course of 2 weeks or so. This is to keep your body safe and ensure that you're not too sore, so that you will enjoy the workouts. Fun and enjoyment is key when it comes to long-term working out!

Body part	Exercise 1	Exercise 2
Legs	Wide-foot squat	Full/half-squat combination
Chest	Press-up	Front press
Back	Dead lift	Bent-over row reverse grip
Shoulders	Reverse press	Upright row
Arms	Full/half bicep combination	Tricep press behind neck
Stomach	Leg crossover	Straight-leg raise
Hips	Front side leg raise	Rear side leg raise

Glossary

Wide-foot squat

The best way to target the soft tissue on the inside of your legs!

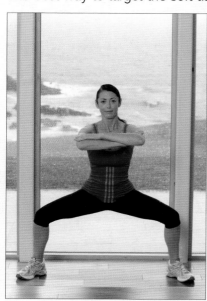
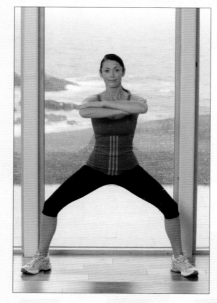

1. Place your feet very wide apart and turn your feet out facing away from the body. This is the key component!

2. Lower yourself as far as feels comfortable and hold.

3. From there simply lower your bum up and down about 3–4 inches towards the floor. There is very little movement in this exercise. That's what makes it so hard.

4. Return to the starting position.

Full/half squat combination

Following on from the normal squat, this combination is a great way to shape up your legs.

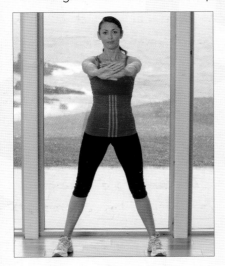 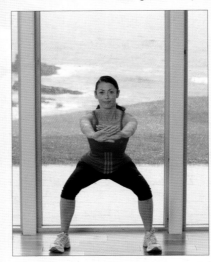

1. Stand with your feet shoulder-width apart, hands crossed at the front to keep your back straight.

2. Bend your knees as low as you feel comfortable. Many guidelines say 90 degrees but not everyone is the same, go as low as feels comfortable for you.

3. Return to the top.

4. On the last of your 20 reps, hold in the lowest part of the squat.

5. Go halfway up and back down 20 times. Feel the burn!

6. Return to the starting position.

This exercise is tough but will give you great legs.

Press-up

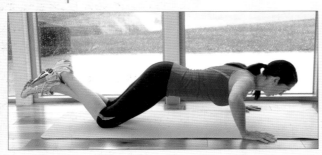 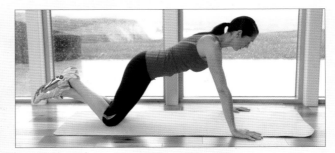

One of the best overall upper-body exercises that there is! There are two versions. Start with the basic version and progress into the harder version.

1. Kneel on your mat.

2. Place your hands on the mat slightly wider than shoulder-width apart and at shoulder level.

3. Place your knees so that your back is parallel to the floor and there should be a 45 degree angle through your hips.

4. Lower your chest to the mat and raise it back up. You should have no back pain at all with this exercise.

If this is too easy, progress into the full press-up, which is the same as the exercise above except that your legs are off the floor. The essential point to note is that your back is flat all the way through. Never, ever arch your back in a press-up.

Real Results

Front press

Now its time to hit the upper body.

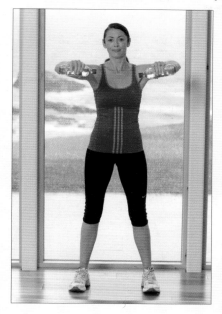 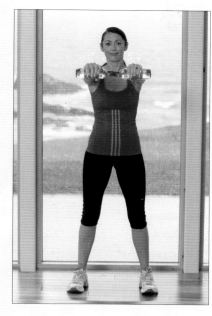

1. Stand with your feet shoulder-width apart, this is essential for good balance, holding the weights by your side.

2. Bring the weights up to your chest at shoulder level.

3. Push them forward out in front of you, keeping your arms at shoulder level all the way through. If you get neck pain here then simply don't lock your arms fully.

4. Return to the starting position.

Dead lift

These are great for your hamstrings and bum, as well as your lower back.

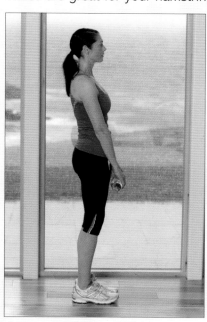 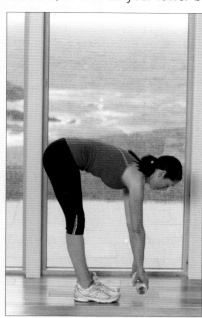

1. Begin by standing with your feet together and your back straight, holding the weights at your hips with your arms nice and relaxed.

2. Keeping your eyes looking straight ahead if possible, lower the weights towards the floor by leaning your body gently forwards towards the floor. Keep your legs as straight as you can, just simply tilt your upper body towards the floor.

3. Return to standing position.

It's essential here to never bounce. It should be a controlled motion and only go as low as you feel comfortable, don't overdo it. Try to keep your legs as straight as possible on the way down.

Bent-over row reverse grip

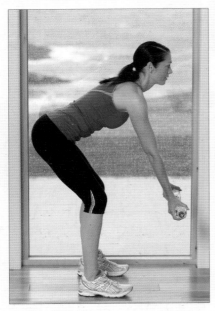 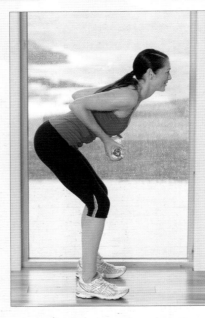

1. Place your feet wide apart.

2. Bend your knees as if you were sitting into a chair.

3. Tilt your upper body forwards so that your back is straight.

4. Extend your arms fully towards the floor, keeping your hands with your palms facing away from the body.

5. Pull up your arms towards your body so that the elbows are higher or in line with your shoulders. Ensure that your arms are extended fully towards the floor to get the best workout.

6. Return to the starting position.

Reverse press

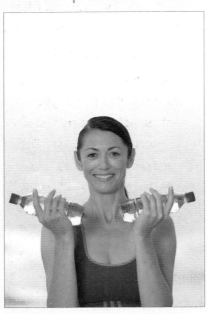 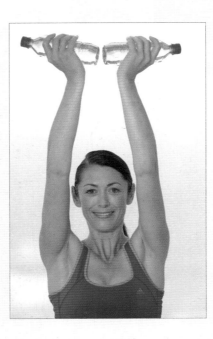

1. Stand with your feet shoulder-width apart, your back straight, holding the weights by your side.

2. Bring the weights to your chest, your palms facing towards you.

3. Extend your arms fully toward the ceiling.

4. Return the weights to your chest. Ensure to keep your arms tucked in at all times.

Upright row

This is one of the best ways to straighten up your posture, by strengthening all the muscles at the back of your neck and shoulders.

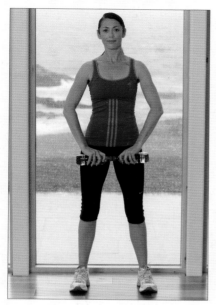
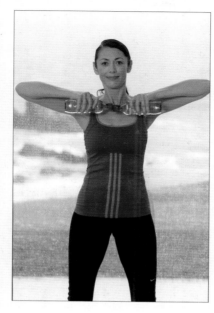

1. Stand tall with your feet shoulder-width apart, holding the weights by your sides.

2. Hold the weights in front of you with your arms fully extended.

3. Raise the weights, moving your elbows first, to your chin (your elbows will be above your shoulders).

4. Return to the starting position.

Full/half bicep combination

This simple combination will give you great shape to the biceps at the front of your arms.

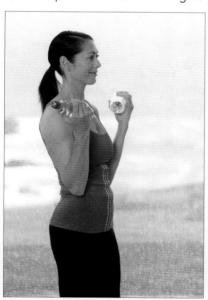
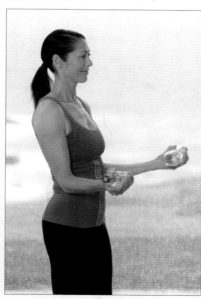

1. Stand straight with your feet shoulder-width apart, holding the weights by your sides.

2. Curl the weights up towards your shoulders with your palms facing towards you, and return back down. The important thing here is to keep your elbows close by your sides, don't let them move away from your body as this means you aren't getting the most from this exercise.

3. When you have done your 20 full curls, restrict the movement and go all the way down but only halfway up. This places more stress on your arms, especially on the lower part of the biceps, which is often neglected.

4. Return to the starting position.

Tricep press behind neck

If the tricep dips are too easy for you, this is the next exercise to target those bingo wings.

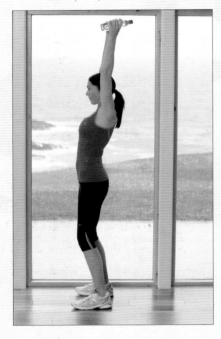 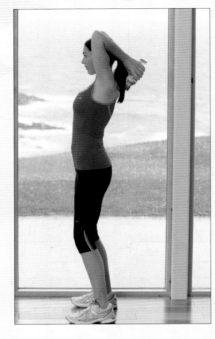

1. Sit or stand with your feet shoulder-width apart, holding the weights by your sides.

2. Raise the weights above your head, with your elbows next to your ears – this is important, as the more your elbows move from your head the less work your triceps actually do.

3. Lower the weights behind your head to the base of your neck.

4. Extend the weight back to the start position. Watch those elbows!

Leg crossover

This is a simple and effective exercise for the pelvis and abdominals.

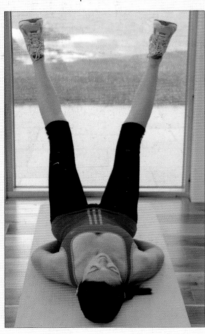 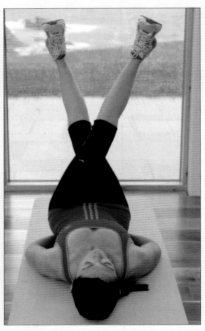

1. Lie on your mat with your hands under your bum, protecting your lower back.

2. Lift your legs outwards at 45 degrees. Ensure to go nice and wide to get the best workout

3. Cross your legs over one another.

4. Repeat the movement 20 times.

As always, the lower your legs are, the harder it will be on the lower back, so don't go too low in the beginning.

Straight-leg raise

This is a great exercise for your pelvis and lower abdominal muscles.

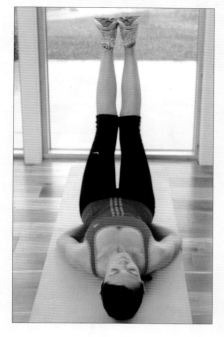 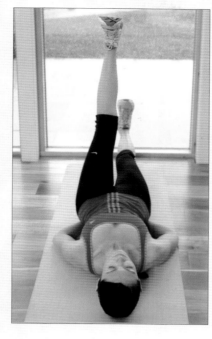

1. Lie on your back on your mat with your hands under your bum. Having your hands under your bum ensures that your lower back stays protected.

2. Raise your legs in the air at roughly 45 degrees.

3. Lift your legs up and down one at a time. The lower your legs go the more work the lower back has to do, so be careful not to go too low with the legs in the beginning.

Front side leg raise

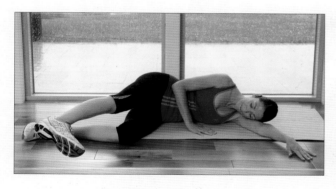 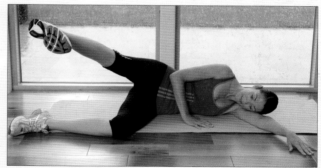

1. Lie on your left side on the mat, ensuring all your joints are in one line. Your shoulders, hips, knees and ankles should all be in a straight line.

2. From there, point your toes towards your face and roll your hip to the front. This is the trick, as it engages your hips/bum to work harder. Watch your hip, always keep it rolled slightly frontwards.

3. Bring your left leg to a 45 degree angle in front of you. This is the angle I want you to keep your leg in for the whole exercise.

4. Raise your right leg in a controlled manner as far up as you feel comfortable.

5. When you have completed the reps, return to the starting position.

6. Repeat the exercise lying on your right side and raising your left leg.

Rear side leg raise

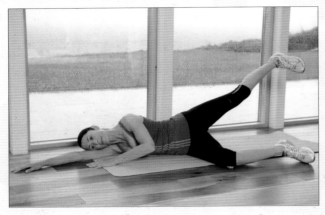 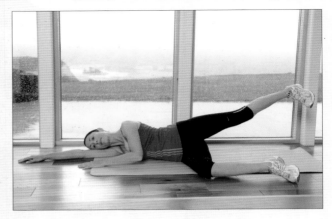

1. Lie on your left side on the mat, ensuring all your joints are in one line. Your shoulders, hips, knees and ankles should all be in a straight line.

2. Point your toes towards your face and roll your hip to the front. This is the trick, as it engages your hips/bum to work harder. Watch your hip, always keep it rolled slightly frontwards.

3. Bring your left leg to a 45 degree angle behind your body. This is the angle I want you to keep your leg for the whole exercise.

4. Raise your right leg in a controlled manner as far up as you feel comfortable.

5. When you have completed the reps, return to the starting position.

6. Repeat the exercise lying on your right side and raising your left leg.

Real Results

Advanced

Are you ready for a tougher workout? Want to challenge yourself even more? Well, this workout will provide that toughness. In the comfort of your own home, this workout will push your body like never before, you will discover muscles that you never knew you had!

Attempt this workout if you consider yourself fit or if you have built yourself up to this using the previous two workouts. This will ensure that you are fit enough and strong enough to attempt these exercises. Start with 1 set in session 1 and build it up over the coming weeks to 3 sets at your own pace, these exercises are designed to sculpt the body and tone it like never before and you will enjoy the challenge of the exercises.

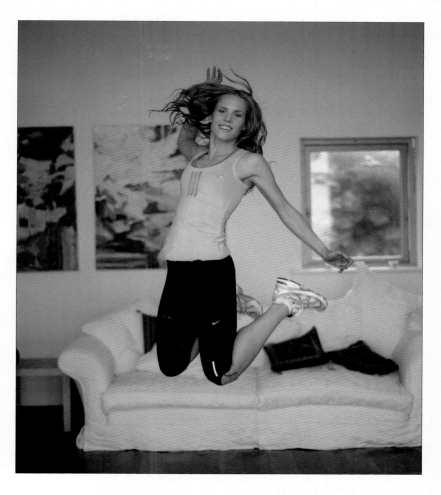

Body part	Exercise 1	Exercise 2
Legs	Three-phase squat	Raised-calf ski squat
Chest	Wide-grip press-up	Straight-arm pec deck
Back	Bent-over row combination	Advanced arm row
Shoulders	Shoulder circle combination	Front raise
Arms	Bicep combination	Advanced tricep extension
Stomach	Bridge/side bridge	Six-pack combination
Hips	Side leg raises full/half	Side leg raise circles

Making the workouts tougher

On the off-chance that you are finding your workouts too easy, there are some really simple ways to make them harder. Try some of these methods.

Heavier resistance Simply choose slightly heavier dumbbells or water bottles and try the same workout to see just what a huge difference it makes. Remember you should be struggling on the last 2 reps of each set, if you're struggling earlier than that, the weights are too heavy. Why not use the slightly heavier weights on the first set and then use your normal ones on the second and third set? Gradually build up to doing the 3 sets with the heavier weights.

Choose your favourite exercises If you have gone through the three routines and now fancy something different, then why not compile your own workout using your favourite exercises? Simply stick to the same method — two exercises per body part so that all body parts get a great workout and aim to get 3 sets done. You can also pick some new exercises from my favourite exercise section on pages 176-179. Choose the exercises for the body part you want to work.

Time If the workout is a little easy, why not put yourself against the clock? Time your workouts and try to beat them the next time that you do that session. The important element is that you don't sacrifice the form of the exercise for pure speed. You will be amazed at just how much tougher the session becomes when you are working towards a time specific goal.

Do some cardiovascular work between sets This is something I use with many of my clients when I do boot camps. In between each set, add a consistent cardiovascular exercise, such as a run around the block, or 5 sets of stair runs. This will not only make the session harder, it will help elevate your heart rate, burning more calories too! It breaks up the session for you mentally too.

Holding movements This is one of the easiest ways to instantly make an exercise harder and improve your workout, without any equipment whatsoever. By holding a movement, you are increasing the workload placed upon the muscle, forcing it to work 50-60 per cent harder than it was working before. You are also taking all the strength from the muscle group, making what was a very easy exercise suddenly quite hard. Simply hold for 30 seconds at the end of each set and you will see just how tough it can make the exercise, you will literally be able to feel the muscle working as the burn in the area increases. As you get stronger you can hold for longer, but start with 30 seconds. Holding movements are particularly effective with exercises that work the hips and bum area, providing a great way of toning up the muscles in those areas.

Glossary

Three-phase squat

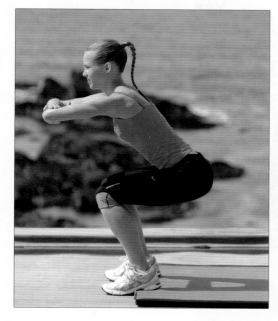 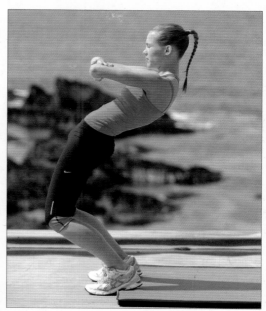

This exercise is a Henry special! It has been passed from Vince's gym, to my dad and finally to me. By putting it in this book, I am giving it to the nation, the ultimate exercise to strengthen and shape your legs.

For this exercise, you will need a block or a book to put your heels on. This emphasises the workload put on the quads and makes them work harder! There are 2 parts to the exercise. Ensure that you conquer part 1 before trying part 2.

1. Begin with your feet on the block, your hands crossed at the front of your body and your back straight.

2. Bend your knees into a normal squat but go as low as possible – bum to your heels if you can.

3. Push your pelvis away from you and then return to the top. Each movement should be done in a controlled motion, don't rush it!

4. Repeat the movement 20 times before returning to the start position.

When you have mastered the first part, it is now time for the second.

Start just as in the first part and squat deeply, heels to bum. Push your pelvis out and return your heels to your bum. You never get to lock out the legs, so they never get to recover, this results in the burning that you feel. It's a tough movement but, believe me, the results will be well worth it!

Raised-calf ski-squat

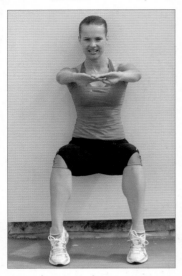

Old school and hard, this great exercise can be done anywhere! All you need is a wall, it really is that simple.

1. Stand with you back against a wall, your feet out in front, shoulder-width apart.

2. Slide your back down so that your quads are parallel to the ground.

3. Raise your feet up on to your tippy toes, and feel the burn! Hold for as long as you can, 30 seconds to 1 minute is good going for this exercise, but, with practise, you will get stronger!

4. Return to the starting position.

Wide-grip press-up

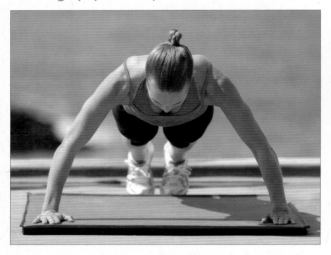 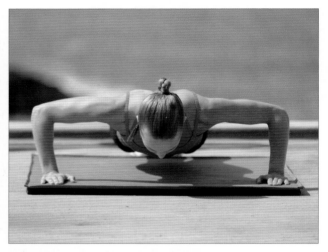

As with the normal press-up, there are two versions. Start with the basic version and progress on to the harder version. The basic version is done with your knees on the mat.

1. Kneel on your mat.

2. Place your hands slightly wider than shoulder-width apart and at shoulder level.

3. Place your knees so that your back is parallel to the floor and there should be a 45 degree angle through your hips.

4. Lower your chest to the mat and come back up. You should have no back pain at all with this exercise.

If this is too easy, then progress into the full press-up. It's the same as the above exercise except that your legs are off the floor. The essential point to note is that your back is flat all the way through. Never ever arch your back with a press-up.

Straight-arm pec deck

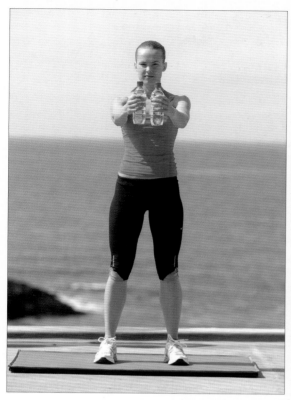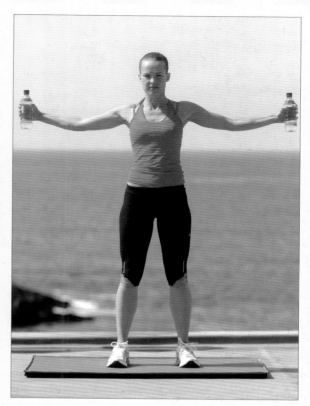

This is a much harder version of the normal pec deck.

1. Stand with your feet shoulder-width apart.

2. Raise your arms straight out to the side in line with your shoulders.

3. Bring your arms to the front of your body so your fingers touch.

4. Move your arms back out the side, keeping your arms straight. If you begin to get neck pain, then slightly bend your arms as this will take the pressure from your neck.

Bent-over row combination

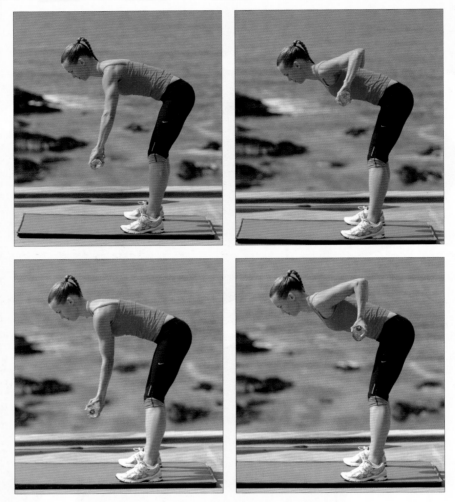

This time, we combine the two exercises to get the ultimate upper-back workout.

1. Place your feet wide apart and bend your knees as if you were sitting into a chair.

2. Tilt your upper body forward so that your back is straight.

3. Extend your arms fully towards the floor, keeping your hands with your palms facing *towards* your body.

4. Pull your arms up towards your body so that your elbows are higher or in line with your shoulders. Ensure that your arms are extended fully towards the floor.

5. Repeat 20 times.

Go straight into the bent over row reverse grip.

6. Extend your arms fully towards the floor, keeping your hands with your palms facing *away from* your body this time.

7. Pull up your arms towards the body so that the elbows are higher or in line with your shoulders. Ensure that your arms are extended fully towards the floor to get the best workout.

8. Repeat 20 times.

Real Results

Advanced arm row

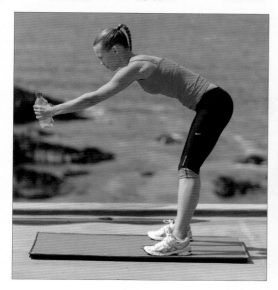 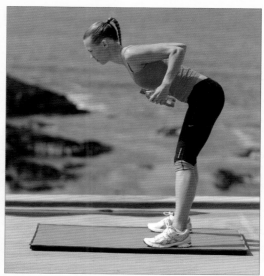

This exercise will give you definition to your back. It is a tougher version of the normal single arm row, there is one simple change, the angle of the movement.

1. Place your feet shoulder-width apart, bend your knees and keep the back straight.

2. Extend your arms to the front at 45 degrees, as if you are sawing a piece of wood, and then raise your arms as high as you feel comfortable, keeping the elbow close by your body. Make sure that you extend the arm fully to the front, getting a full stretch. By changing the angle of the movement you will give shape on your back like never before!

Shoulder circle combination

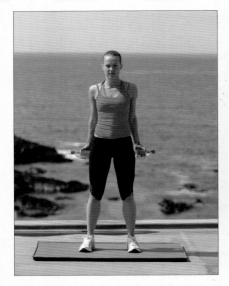
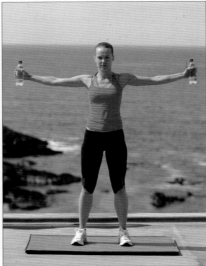
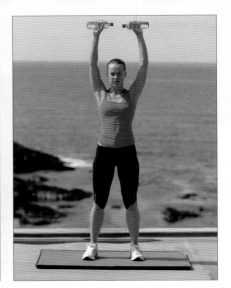

Think toned, defined shoulders, firm and shapely. This exercise is one of the secrets to getting the shoulders that you always wanted. There are 4 parts to this exercise.

1. With the weights in your hands, stand with your feet shoulder-width apart and a straight posture.
2. Start with the weights behind your back, palms facing your bum.
3. Keeping your arms straight, create a full circle, meeting the weights at the top above your head.
4. Repeat this movement 20 times.
5. On the last circle, hold the weights at the top.

From there, part 2 is a top-half movement.

6. Bring the weights to shoulder level.
7. Take them back to the top.
8. Repeat this movement 20 times, ending with the weights at shoulder level.

The third part of this exercise is for the bottom half.

9. Straighten your arms to bring the weights down to your hips.
10. Bring the weights halfway up.
11. Repeat this movement 20 times, ending with the weights by your hips.

Now the final part.

12. Repeat the first four steps of this exercise, completing 20 full circles.

This will burn like hell, you will feel your shoulders working hard during this movement and that's the whole idea!

Front raise

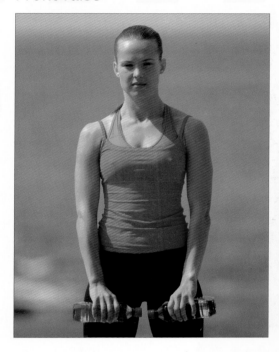 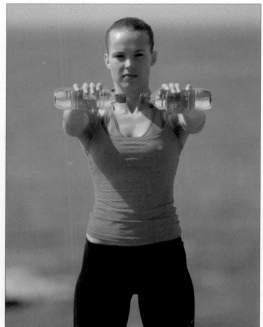

This is one of the best ways to target the muscles across the back of your neck. Those muscles that look so good in a dress or a shirt when they are toned.

1. Begin with the feet shoulder-width apart, holding the weights in front of your body at your hips, palms facing towards your body. The weights should be about 2 inches away from you so that they aren't touching your body.

2. Keeping your arms straight, raise the weights up to eye level and back to the starting position.

The reason that this exercise becomes hard is the fact that the weights never touch your body, and so your muscles are never allowed to rest. Be careful not to arch your back, always keep it straight.

Bicep combination

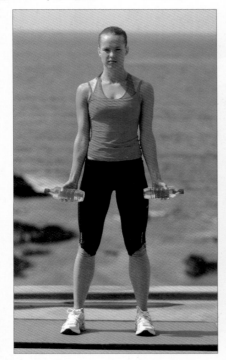 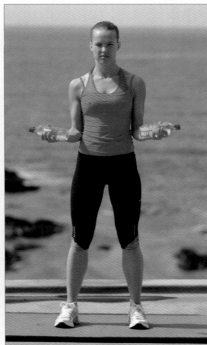 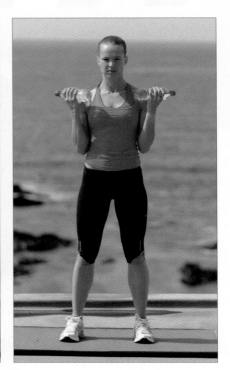

There are three sections to this amazing combination.

1. Stand straight with your feet shoulder-width apart, arms fully extended towards the floor, holding the weights.

2. Curl the weights up towards your shoulder and return back down.

The important thing here is to keep your elbows close by your side, don't let them move away from the body as this means you aren't getting the most from the exercise.

3. Repeat this movement twenty times and return to the starting position.

Now for the second section.

4. Repeat the exercise as in the first section but restrict the movement and go all the way down but only halfway up.

This places more stress on the arms, especially on the lower part of the arm.

5. Repeat this movement twenty times and return to the starting position.

Now for the third part.

6. Holding the weights and with your arms by your sides, turn the palms of your hands to face your body.

7. Curl the weights up towards you and twist on the way up, so that the palms are facing you by the time the curl comes to the top of the arm.

8. Repeat twenty times and return to the starting position.

Real Results

Advanced tricep extension

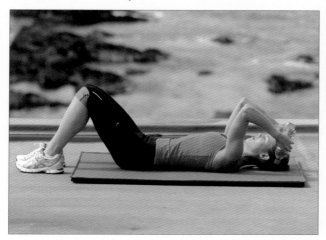 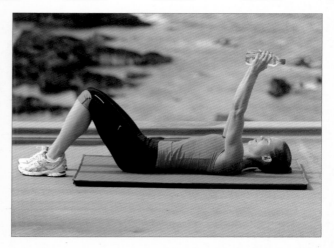

By now, you should have firm toned arms, from all of the tricep exercises so far. This exercise is a more advanced movement, targeting the tricep muscle in a slightly different way.

1. Lie on your mat, holding the weights to either side of your face.

2. Extend the weights at 45 degrees away from your body (rather than straight up to the ceiling).

Keep the movement controlled at all times and squeeze the tricep on the extension to get the full benefits from the movement.

Bridge/side bridge

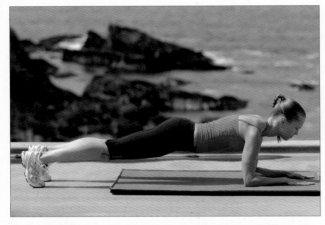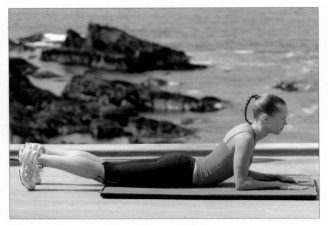

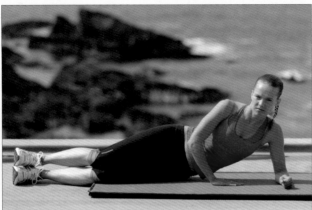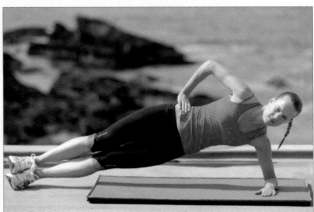

There are 2 parts to this exercise. Start with full bridge and progress into the side bridge.

1. Lie on your front on the mat and place your elbows at shoulder level, keeping your back parallel to the floor.

2. Keeping your legs straight, raise your stomach off the mat keeping your back parallel to the floor.

3. Suck your belly button towards your spine and hold for 30 seconds initially – increase to 1 minute as you get stronger.

Ensure that there is no dip in your back whatsoever. If you have any back pain, stop straight away.

Next go into your side bridge.

4. Turn onto your left side on the mat, leaning on your left elbow.

5. Raise your whole body off the mat, with your feet and elbow being the two points of contact with the mat.

6. Keeping your shoulders in line and your legs straight hold this position for 30 seconds initially and then build up to 1 minute.

7. Repeat for your right side.

Six-pack combination

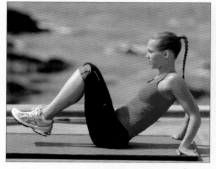
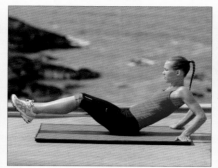
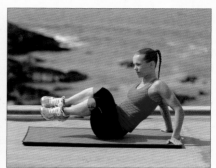
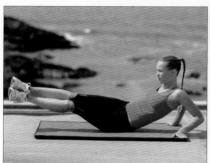
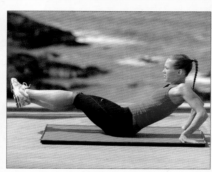
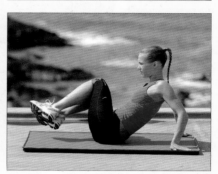

We all want a firm flatter stomach, no doubt about it. This is one of my favourite exercises as it works all the muscles around the stomach area, the sides of your waist and your pelvic muscles too, giving what I believe is the ultimate workout for the stomach area. Like many of the advanced exercises, there are 4 parts to this exercise.

1. Sit on the mat with your hands behind your body and legs out in front.
2. Bring your knees up to meet your body and, keeping your feet raised off the floor, extend your legs away from your body. While your legs are coming in, your body also comes in to meet them.

Part 2 is to do the very same movement, but focusing on your right side.

3. Rotate your body onto your right hip.
4. Repeat the movement as above.

Part 3 is to focus on your left side.

5. Rotating onto your left hip.
6. Repeat the movement.

Part 4 is the same as the first – focus back on the centre.

7. Repeat steps 1 and 2.
8. Return to the starting position.

The important point of this exercise is that the feet never touch the ground, always try to keep them up in the air so your body doesn't get time to recover. As with any exercise, if you get back pain then stop straight away!

The Exercises

Side leg raises full/half combination

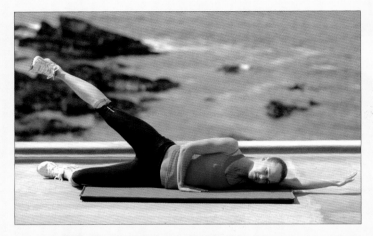

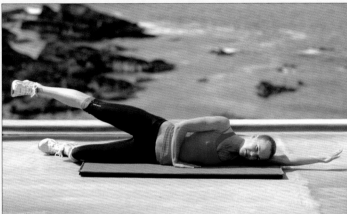

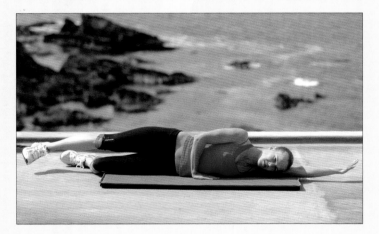

A tough but brilliant combination to transform your bum and hips.

1. Lie on your left side on the mat, ensuring all your joints are in line. Your shoulders, hips, knees and ankles should all be in a straight line.

2. Point your toes towards your face and roll your hip to the front. This is the trick, as it engages your hips/bum to work harder. Watch that hip, always keep it rolled slightly frontwards.

3. Raise your right leg in a controlled manner as far up as you feel comfortable and repeat 20 times.

4. On the final lift, hold your leg at halfway down.

5. Repeat the movement 20 times from the halfway point up.

6. On the final lift, hold your leg at the halfway point.

7. Repeat the movement 20 times from the halfway point down.

8. Repeat lying on your right side using your left leg.

Feel the burn!

Side leg raise circle

1. Lie on your left side on the mat, ensuring all your joints are in one line. Your shoulders, hips, knees and ankles should all be in a straight line.

2. Point the toes towards your face and roll your hip to the front. This is the trick, as it engages your hips/bum to work harder. Watch that hip, always keep it rolled slightly frontwards.

3. Raise your right leg and hold it halfway.

4. Rotate your leg in a circular motion clockwise 20 times.

5. Rotate your leg anti-clockwise 20 times.

6. Repeat lying on your right side using your left leg.

This is an effective, old-school Pilates exercise that works so well!

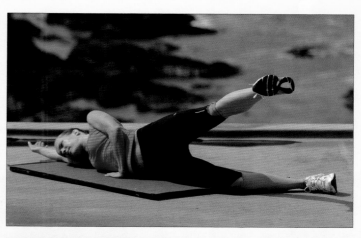

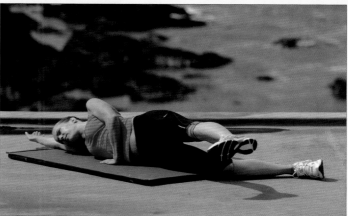

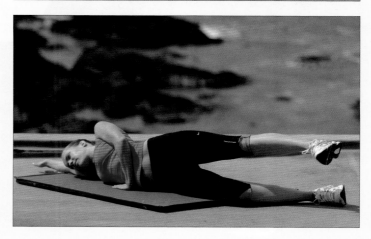

Karl's favourite exercises

These are just a few of my favourite exercises that I use with clients and that I use in my own training. You can substitute these into the routines above or even add them in as extras. They tend to be slightly more advanced, so I wouldn't recommend them for beginners, but they are fantastic exercises that will seriously challenge you. One of the important elements to all workouts is that you feel challenged. This will help to keep you interested so that you keep training, boredom can stop even the most committed person from training. So try a few of these, but remember they are for the advanced!

Chin-up

The oldest exercise going! In many people's view, myself included, chin-ups are one of the best exercises that exist! For your arms, back, triceps, waist, core, pelvis, you name it, nearly every muscle group can be worked by changing your position on the bar.

Men and women alike are often intimidated by chin-ups, because they can't do as many as other people they see using the bar. Well here is the good news, the only

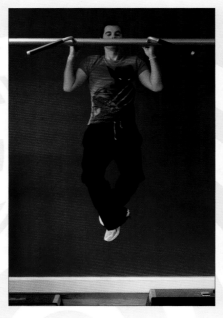
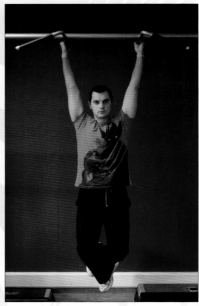

way to get better at chin-ups is by repetition. Simply by doing a few sets of as many as you can, you will get better and better. Make sure that you extend your arms fully on the way down, ensuring that you give your arms the workout they deserve.

When starting off, do negative chin-ups to build up strength. By this I mean jump up, touching your chest off the bar and then lower yourself to the ground in a controlled way for 5 seconds. This will help to build up the strength in your arms.

When doing chin-ups, you can vary the muscles that you work by changing your hand position.

Hand position	Body part worked
Regular grip	All bicep
Wide grip	Inner bicep
Close grip	Outer bicep
Reverse grip	Forearms/tricep/bicep

Bench crossover

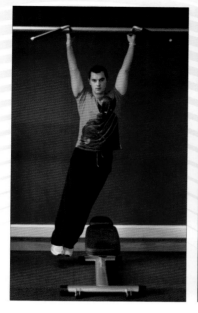 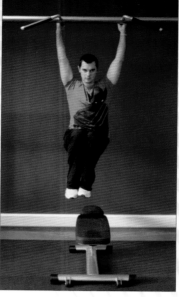 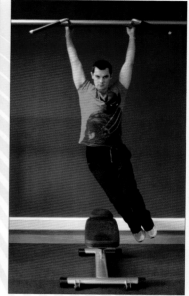

This is one of my favourite ab exercises but can really only be done in a gym environment. You need a bench, and sometimes arm supports if you find your arms get tired hanging from the bar. Place the bench below the position your feet drop to when you are in position on the bar. Hanging from the bar, extend your legs to the left of the bench, then bend your knees and raise them to your chest as you cross over the bench, then extend your legs to the right of the bench. Always go all the way down with the legs and remember that over and back counts as one rep. This is one of the ultimate exercises to sculpt the stomach area, it's not easy but, sure, the best ones aren't.

Jump squat

Jump squats are a great cardiovascular workout combined with a great way to sculpt your legs. The technique is easy but they are hard, be warned! The essential part is to ensure that your feet are wide enough apart and that you go as low as you can on the way down. Simply start wide on the feet, then touch the floor with your hands, bum to ankles and then jump as high and explosively as you can, on the way down go straight into the next rep, no stopping!

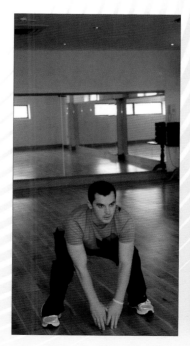 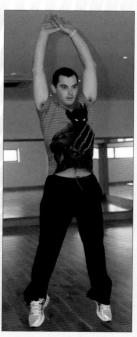

Bench jump

Another explosive movement, great for shaping a fit pair of legs and providing a tough cardiovascular movement too. Start with your body in front of a bench or step. Bend your elbows slightly in front of you, then bend from your hips and explosively jump up onto the bench in front of you returning to ground. Return to the starting position and then go again.

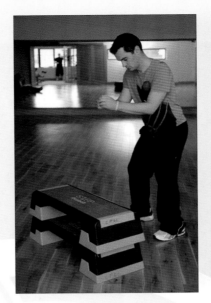
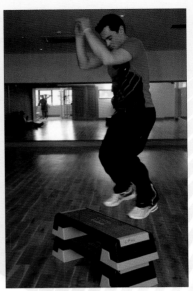

Wide-grip chin-up

One of my favourite back exercises, this will widen and sculpt your pack like very little else, and also provide a great arm workout in general. Place your hands wide on the bar, ensuring you extend your arms fully. Raise yourself so that you touch your chest off the bar and extend your arms back down. Most people don't extend their arms on the way down, and so don't get the best benefits from the exercise, or they rock their body on the way up. Try to keep the body controlled so that your arms and back do all the work!

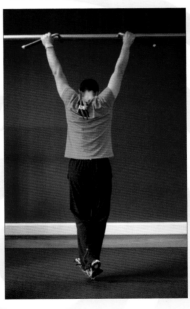
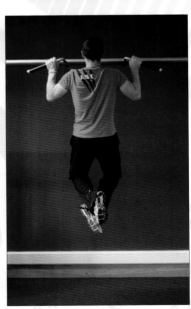

Assisted leg press

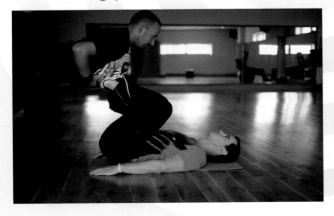
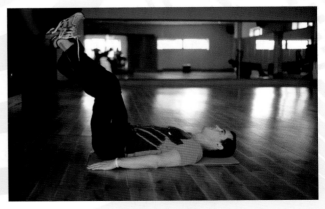

Real Results

I love doing this exercise with my clients as it is such a great leg workout for the hamstrings and the quads. I know it looks kind of scary, but watch those legs transform from doing it! You obviously need a friend to help you with this one! Keeping your back flat on the mat, place your feet on the chest of who ever is helping you, lower your legs close to your chest and then extend the legs back up, ensuring not to lock them out. By locking them out you will make it easier for the legs, so only lock them 80 per cent of the way.

Squat and circle

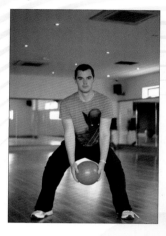 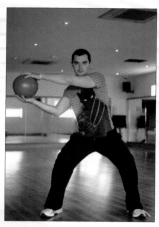 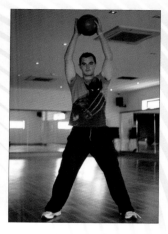 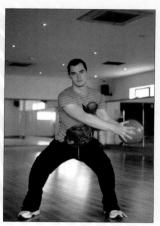

A brilliant all-over body exercise, this is one of the staples of my sessions with my clients. It works the legs and upper body, making the inside of the legs and the waist do a huge amount of work. Stand with your feet wider than shoulder-width apart, holding a weight in front of you. Now keeping your hands together holding the weight, squat and make a circular motion with your arms, drawing the full 360 degrees! As you raise the weight above your head, stand up and lower to a squat position again as you bring the weight back to the starting position. Do 20 in a clockwise direction and 20 in an anti-clockwise direction.

Close-grip wall press-up

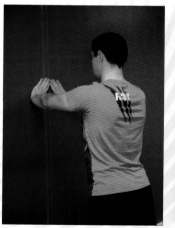 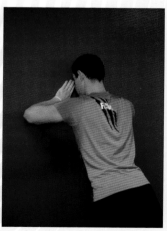

Often, women tell me that they can't do press-ups, this exercise is one that I use with them as a variant to a traditional floor press-up. It is for the triceps at the back of the arm and is so effective yet so simple to do. Stand around 2 feet away from a wall, with your feet shoulder-width apart. Your hands should be at the nipple line and close together so that you form a triangle with your thumbs and your index finger. That's the key part, forcing your triceps to do all the work. Lower your body towards the wall and press your arms back out. Your arms will naturally move away from the body in a bow-like motion on the way in, this is exactly the idea! Wall press-ups can be done several ways with different hand positions to work different body parts, the important thing with all of them is that your back never arches in, it should always be nice and straight!

A quick summary... beginners

Photocopy this page and refer to it whilst doing your workout.

Squat (p159) ❶ Stand with your feet shoulder-width apart. ❷ Cross your hands at the front to keep your back straight. ❸ Bend your knees as low as you feel comfortable. ❹ Return to the top.

Lunge (p159) ❶ Stand with your feet together, your posture straight. ❷ Lunge forward with your right leg, bending your left knee towards the floor. ❸ Return to an upright position. ❹ Repeat with your left leg.

Pec deck (p160) ❶ Stand with your feet shoulder-width apart. ❷ Raise your elbows in front of you to 90 degrees in line with your shoulders. ❸ Try to touch your elbows together in front of your body. ❹ Lower your elbows.

Bench press (p160) ❶ Lie on your back on your mat with your knees bent. ❷ With a weight in either hand, extend your arms directly above your nipple line. ❸ Lower your elbows to the floor in line with your shoulders.

 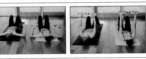

Single-arm row (p161) ❶ Place one knee on a chair or bench. ❷ Place your hand on a chair. ❸ Extend your right arm to the floor and raise your left arm. Keep your elbow close by your body. Extend your arm fully on the way down. ❹ Return to an upright position. ❺ Repeat with left arm.

Bent-over row (p162) ❶ Stand with your feet wide apart. ❷ Bend your knees as if you were sitting into a chair and tilt your upper body forward so that your back is straight. ❸ Extend your arms fully towards the floor. ❹ Return to an upright position.

Military press (p162) ❶ Place your feet are shoulder-width apart for balance. ❷ Holding the weights at your shoulders. ❸ Press them straight up, touching in the middle. ❹ Return the weights all the way down so that they touch your shoulders.

Side lateral raise (p163) ❶ Place your feet shoulder-width apart. ❷ Hold the weights by your hips, not in front of you. ❸ Raise the weights to the side, with a slight bend in your arms. ❹ Lower the weights back to your hips.

 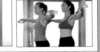

Tricep dip (p163) ❶ Sit on a chair or bench. ❷ Place your hands by your hips and your feet out in front, hamstrings parallel to floor. ❸ Bend your elbows so that your bum goes towards the floor. ❹ Extend your arms so that they are fully locked out.

Bicep curl (p164) ❶ Stand with your feet shoulder-width apart, arms fully extended towards the floor, holding a weight in each hand. ❷ Curl the weights up towards your shoulders, keeping your elbows close by your side. ❸ Return to the starting position.

 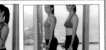

Regular sit-up (p164) ❶ Lie on your back with your knees bent. ❷ Place your hands behind your head, just resting in your hands. ❸ Look at a fixed point on your ceiling. ❹ Sit up about 3–4 inches, using your stomach, not your neck, and return to the floor. If you have any neck pain, stop straight away.

Bridge (p165) ❶ Lie down on the mat on your stomach and place your elbows on the mat, just under your chest. ❷ Keeping your knees at 45 degrees, raise your stomach off the mat keeping your back parallel to the floor. ❸ Suck your belly button towards your spine and hold for 30 seconds.

Side-leg raise (p165) ❶ Lie on your left side on the mat. Your shoulders, hips, knees and ankles should all be in a straight line. ❷ Point your toes towards your face and roll your hip to the front. ❸ Raise and lower your right leg. ❹ Repeat lying on your right side.

Bum kick (p166) ❶ Get onto your mat, on all fours with shoulders and knees body-distant apart. ❷ Bring your right knee into your chest and then extend your leg fully back behind you. ❸ Repeat the exercise using your left leg.

Please note: The above exercises are listed in summary form only to prompt you whilst doing your workout. Check the relevant page for complete instructions for each exercise.

A quick summary... medium

Photocopy this page and refer to it whilst doing your workout.

Wide-foot squat (p153) ❶ With your feet wide apart, turn your feet away from the body. ❷ Lower yourself as far as feels comfortable and hold. ❸ Lower your bum up and down about 3–4 inches towards the floor.

Full/half squat combination (p154) ❶ With your feet shoulder-width apart and hands crossed at the front to keep your back straight, bend your knees as low as you feel comfortable. ❷ Return to the top. ❸ On the last rep hold in the lowest part of the squat. ❹ Go halfway up and back down 20 times.

Press-up (p154) ❶ On your mat, kneel with your hands on the mat slightly wider than shoulder-width apart (at shoulder level) so that your back is parallel to the floor with a 45 degree angle through your hips and knees. ❷ Lower your chest to the mat and raise back up.

Front press (p155) ❶ Stand with your feet shoulder-width apart, holding the weights by your side. ❷ Bring the weights up to your chest at shoulder level. ❸ Push them forward out in front of you, keeping your arms at shoulder level all the way through.

Dead lift (p155) ❶ Standing with your feet together and your back straight hold the weights at your hips with relaxed arms. ❷ Looking straight ahead, lower the weights towards the floor by leaning your body gently forwards. Keep your legs straight, just simply tilt your upper body towards the floor. ❸ Return to standing position.

Bent-over row reverse grip (p156) ❶ Place your feet wide apart and bend your knees as if you were sitting into a chair, your upper body tilted forwards so your back is flat. ❷ With your palms facing away from your body, extend arms fully towards the floor. ❺ Pull up your arms towards your body (your elbows will be higher or in line with your shoulders).

Reverse press (p156) ❶ Stand with your feet shoulder-width apart, your back straight, holding the weights by your side. ❷ Bring the weights to your chest, palms facing towards you. ❸ Extend your arms fully toward the ceiling. ❹ Return the weights to your chest.

Upright row (p157) ❶ Stand with your feet shoulder-width apart, hold the weights with your arms fully extended in front of your body. ❷ Moving your elbows first, raise the weights to your chin (your elbows will be above your shoulders).

Full/half bicep combination (p157) ❶ Stand straight with feet shoulder-width apart, holding weights by your sides. ❷ Curl them up towards your shoulders and return down. ❸ After 20 full curls, restrict the movement, go all the way down but only halfway up.

Tricep press behind neck (p158) ❶ Sit or stand with your feet shoulder-width apart, holding the weights by your sides. ❷ Raise the weights above your head, with your elbows next to your ears. ❸ Lower the weights behind your head to the base of your neck.

Leg crossovers (p158) ❶ Lie on your mat with your hands under your bum, protecting your lower back. ❷ Lift your legs outwards at 45 degrees. ❸ Cross your legs over one another.

Straight-leg raise (p159) ❶ Lie on your back on your mat with your hands under your bum. ❷ Raise your legs in the air at roughly 45 degrees. ❸ Lift your legs up and down one at a time.

Front side leg raise (p159) ❶ Lie on your left side on the mat with all your joints in one line. ❷ Point your toes towards your face, roll your hip to the front and bring your left leg to a 45 degree angle. ❹ Raise your right leg. ❺ Repeat for your left leg.

Rear side leg raise (p160) ❶ Lie on your left side on the mat with all your joints in one line. ❷ Point your toes towards your face and roll your hip to the front. ❸ Bring your left leg to a 45 degree angle behind your body. ❹ Raise your right leg. ❺ Repeat for your left leg.

Please note: The above exercises are listed in summary form only to prompt you whilst doing your workout. Check the relevant page for complete instructions for each exercise.

A quick summary... advanced

Photocopy this page and refer to it whilst doing your workout.

Three-phase squat (p163) ❶ Standing on a block, your hands crossed at the front of your body and your back straight, bend your knees into a normal squat but go as low as possible. ❷ Push your pelvis away from you and then return to the top. ❸ After twenty reps, squat deeply, heels to bum. Push your pelvis out and return your heels to your bum.

Raised-calf ski-squat (p164) ❶ Stand with you back against a wall with your feet shoulder-width apart. ❷ Slide your back down so that your quads are parallel to the ground. ❸ Raise your feet up on to your tippy toes. Hold for 30 seconds.

Wide-grip press-up (p164) ❶ Kneeling on your mat, place your hands at shoulder level, slightly wider than shoulder-width apart. Your back should be parallel to the floor with a 45 degree angle through your hips. ❷ Lower your chest to the mat and come back up.

Straight-arm pec deck (p165) ❶ Standing with your feet shoulder-width apart, raise your arms out to the side in line with shoulders. ❷ Bring your arms to the front of body so fingers touch. ❹ Move your arms back out the side, keeping your arms straight.

Bent-over row combination (p166) ❶ Feet wide apart, bend knees as if you were sitting into a chair (keep your back straight). ❷ Extend arms fully towards the floor with palms facing away from body. ❹ Pull your arms up towards your body (your elbows will be higher/in line with your shoulders). ❺ Repeat with your palms facing away from your body.

Advanced arm row (p166) ❶ Place your feet shoulder-width apart, bend your knees and keep your back straight. ❷ Extend your arms fully to the front at 45 degrees and raise them as high as is comfortable, keeping the elbow close by your body.

Shoulder circle combination (p168) ❶ Stand with feet shoulder-width apart, weights behind back, palms facing bum. ❷ With straight arms create a full circle, weights above head. ❸ On last circle, hold at top, bring weights to shoulder level. ❹ Return to top and repeat. ❺ Lower weights to hips, bring halfway up and repeat movement. ❻ Repeat first 2 steps.

Front-raise (p169) ❶ With feet shoulder-width apart hold the weights in front of your body at your hips, about 2 inches away from your body. ❷ Keeping your arms straight, raise the weights to eye level lower to the starting position.

Bicep combination (p170) ❶ Feet shoulder-width apart, holding weights, fully extend your arms down. ❷ Curl weights towards your shoulders and return down. ❸ On final rep hold the movement halfway up and repeat from halfway point down. ❺ Weights by your sides, turn the palms of your hands inwards. ❻ Curl weights upwards, twisting palms at top.

Advanced tricep extension (p171) ❶ Lie on your mat, holding the weights to either side of your face. ❷ Extend the weights at 45 degrees away from your body. Squeeze the tricep on the extension to get the full benefits from the movement.

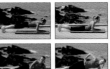

Bridge/side bridge (p172) ❶ Lie on your mat, with your elbows at shoulder level. ❷ Keeping your legs and back straight, raise your stomach off the mat. ❸ Suck your belly button towards your spine and hold for 30 seconds. ❹ Turn onto your left side, leaning on your left elbow. ❺ Raise your whole body, with only your feet and elbow on the mat. ❻ Hold for 30 seconds. ❼ Repeat for your right side.

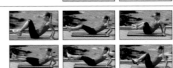

Six-pack combination (p173) ❶ Sitting on the mat with hands behind body and legs in front, bring your knees up to meet your body and, with your feet raised, extend your legs away from your body. ❷ Rotate your body onto your right hip and repeat the movement as above. ❸ Rotating onto your left hip, repeat the movement. ❹ Repeat steps ❶ and ❷.

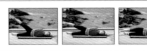

Side leg raise (p174) ❶ Lying on your left side, raise and lower leg 20 times. ❸ On final rep, hold leg halfway down and repeat movement from halfway point up. ❹ On final lift, hold leg at halfway point and repeat down. ❺ Repeat for left leg.

Side leg raise circle (p175) ❶ Lying on left side, point toes towards your face and roll your hip to the front. ❷ Raise right leg and hold it halfway. ❸ Rotate your leg in a circular motion clockwise 20 times and anti-clockwise 20 times. ❹ Repeat for your left leg.

Please note: The above exercises are listed in summary form only to prompt you whilst doing your workout. Check the relevant page for complete instructions for each exercise.

Long-distance endurance events

Are you ready?

If you have your set your sights on a marathon, an ironman or any long-distance endurance event, there are many different elements that you need to consider before you register.

▶ **Time:** Although the event may look incredible, do you have the time to train for it? Remember that training plans for endurance events can take anything from 7 to 20 hours per week, that's a lot of training! Do you have time to get that training done?

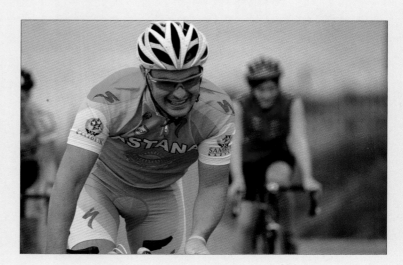

▶ **Support of loved ones:** In your quest for that life-changing event, sit down and discuss it with your partner and friends. All the training you need to do will affect, and put a strain on, your relationships. You won't have the energy to go to all those parties and nights out that you used to, it's a big sacrifice and your partner may have to take on more in terms of looking after children or housework. So make sure that you have their support.

▶ **Training plan or coach:** This is essential. I have learned first hand that these events need a structured training plan devised by professionals who know what they are doing. Just because your friend used a certain training plan doesn't mean that that plan will work for you. For marathons, generic training plans can work reasonably well but when you begin to go longer than that, you will need to get the advice of a coach. There are many out there, both in Ireland and online. Check out their experience within the sport you are doing and also their results with other clients. I use a European coach to whom I chat once a week on Skype and he sends me my training plans on a monthly basis.

▶ **Race choice:** It is essential that you choose the best race possible for you. There are so many things to take into consideration, distance, travel time, support, temperature, course and reputation. If you don't like the heat, then it makes sense not to choose a race that takes place in the Sahara Desert! The distance of endurance races is what provides the initial challenge, after that, you can increase the challenge by choosing a more difficult course or hotter country. But if it's your first one, try to choose a race that is suited to first timers.

Getting started

When you've decided that you are ready to enter an event, it's necessary to think about how you approach and train for your race — and what you shouldn't do.

Nutrition

When you increase your training for an endurance event, you will need to monitor your food more carefully. It's easy to think that because you are training so much, you can eat what you want, but you need to ensure that you are helping your body to recover and fuelling yourself for your next workout. Always start with a large carbohydrate meal in the morning, this will help to give you energy throughout the day!

Pre-training take a sugar-based product for a little energy kick to get your body started if you feel tired. During the training, aim to drink every 15 to 20 minutes and eat every 30 minutes. Post-training aim to eat/drink within 20 minutes for optimum recovery. If your sessions are over 1 hour in duration, I would recommend taking some salt/electrolyte tablets to prevent dehydration and cramp.

Time	Type of food	Example
Pre-training	Sugar/caffine	Jaffa cakes, coffee
During training	Easily absorbed calories	Chocolate
Post-training	Ratio of 4:1, carbs to protein	Ensure, Yazoo

Carb loading

There are three main methods of carb loading on the market. The whole idea of carb loading is to pre-fuel the body for the race ahead.

Type	Method	Foods	Era	Theory
Full-week load	Increased carb intake, 7 days before race	Pasta, bread, rice, potatoes	Old school	Increased glycogen into the muscles
2-day load	Increased carb intake, 2 days before race	Pasta, bread, rice, potatoes	Modern	Increased glycogen into the muscles after reducing it for the previous 5 days
Fat load	Increased fat intake 1 day before the race	Dark chocolate, Thai food, creamy sauces	New age	The body has enough carbs from reduced training and runs on fat in endurance races

As you can see from the three methods above there are very different styles of pre-race nutrition. I have tried all three, and the fat load method is my current preference.

Overtraining

This is one of the most common mistakes that endurance athletes make, myself included. If you overtrain without backing off, then you risk blowing your whole race – believe me, I have done it. Overtraining syndrome generally occurs in athletes who train beyond their body's ability to recover. When training for an endurance event, you train long distances and put in a huge number of hours, often combined with a several other commitments. Without adequate rest and recovery, these long training hours can backfire and actually decrease performance as your body doesn't have time to recover. For me, it was like a fuse blowing. I was cycling with some friends one day and all of a sudden I had no power, fuse blown!

Common warning signs of overtraining include:

▸ Washed-out feeling, tired, drained, lack of energy.

▸ Mild-leg soreness, general aches and pains that don't go away after a few days.

▸ Pain in muscles and joints.

▸ Sudden drop in performance.

▸ Insomnia.

▸ Headaches.

▸ Decreased immunity (increased number of colds and sore throats).

▸ Decrease in training capacity/intensity.

▸ Moodiness and irritability.

▸ Depression.

▸ Loss of enthusiasm for the sport.

▸ Decreased appetite.

▸ Increased incidence of injuries.

▸ A need to exercise.

▸ In extreme circumstances even hay-fever-like symptoms.

If you think you are overtraining, the first thing to do is reduce or stop your exercise and take a few days rest. The general rule is the longer the overtraining has occurred for, the more rest that is required. Therefore, early detection is very important. If the overtraining has only occurred for a short period of time (e.g. 3 to 4 weeks), then not training for 3 to 5 days is usually sufficient rest. Drink plenty of fluids and alter your diet if necessary. Sometimes, you will need to increase your food intake to get the required nutrients into your body. A sports massage can also help you recharge overused muscles.

After a few days try a light session and see how your body feels. If you still feel very fatigued then stop the session, go home and rest for an extra few days and try the session again. Every body is different and it can be hard to know just how overtrained you are, so trial and error is required.

The intensity of your training can be maintained but the total volume must be lower and you must build it back up gradually or modify it so that you do less training. So if you were running 4 times a week now run twice a week but hold a similar pace. Remember it is essential to lower the volume!

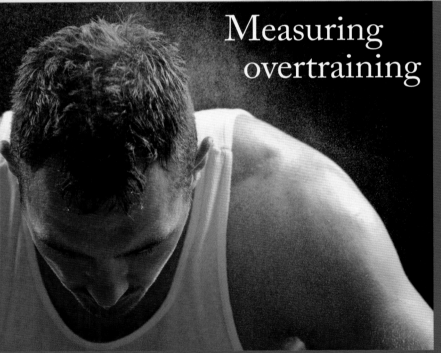

Measuring overtraining

There are several ways you can measure some signs of overtraining:

▷ **Track your heart rate during training.** If it is high and your effort level is low then you may be close to being overtrained.

▷ **Track your resting heart rate each morning.** Any marked increase from the norm may indicate that you aren't fully recovered and you may need more rest.

▷ **Keep a training log that includes a note about how your feel each day.** This can help you notice downward trends and decreased enthusiasm. It's important to listen to your body signals and rest when you feel tired.

While there are many proposed ways to test objectively for overtraining, the most accurate and sensitive measurements are psychological signs and symptoms and changes in your mental state. Decreased positive feelings for sports and increased negative feelings, such as depression, anger, fatigue and irritability, often appear after a few days of intensive overtraining. You will know your body better than anyone else, if you begin to lose interest in your training and hate going out for the sessions, then, chances are, you're close to being overtrained.

It is important that the factors that led to the overtraining are identified and corrected. Otherwise, the overtraining syndrome is likely to recur. In more severe cases, the training programme may have to be interrupted for weeks, and it may take months to recover. An alternate form of exercise can be substituted to help prevent the exercise withdrawal syndrome but serious rest is required.

The sort of person who signs up for endurance events tend to be high achievers, who find it very hard to step back from the training and actually rest. This is where having a qualified coach makes all the difference, the coach will be able to monitor how you are doing and instruct you as required.

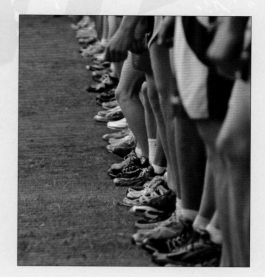

Race-day pointers

I have raced many different endurance events and I am always amazed by the race-day preparation and the difference between those who do well and those who don't – remember, 'Failing to plan is planning to fail.' The longer the race, the more important the planning becomes. You should try to plan for most eventualities just in case they happen.

Here are some easy yet simple tips to improve your race day:

▸ Eat a good, carb-based breakfast, such as porridge.

▸ Eat at least 2 hours before the race.

▸ Try to go to the toilet before you get to the race.

▸ Get there early, the less stress before a race, the better.

▸ Bring an old top with you that you can throw away when you have started.

▸ Vaseline your feet and any other areas that may chaff.

▸ Never race in new runners/clothing, always race in gear that you have trained in.

▸ Have a pre-race plan and stick to it.

▸ Start slow and build up your speed as you find your rhythm.

▸ Ideally try to see the course before the race so that you know where the hills, etc. are. It's much better than getting a surprise that you weren't expecting.

▸ If you are a walker don't start at the front.

▸ If you are beginning to lose focus on the run, a wise man once gave me a great tip: find a nice bum and sit behind it! This tip has been essential in my marathons.

▸ Give yourself mini goals for each kilometre. I use people as mine. Pick someone that you want to be in front of by the next kilometre mark.

▸ Use the crowd to spur you on!

▸ Always aim to finish strong, hence the reason why I recommend starting slow.

Finally, when you've finished – reward yourself! It is essential to have a reward after all your hard work. Mine is garlic chips and a veggie burger (as I am a vegetarian). Your reward will taste all the better after you have worked so hard.

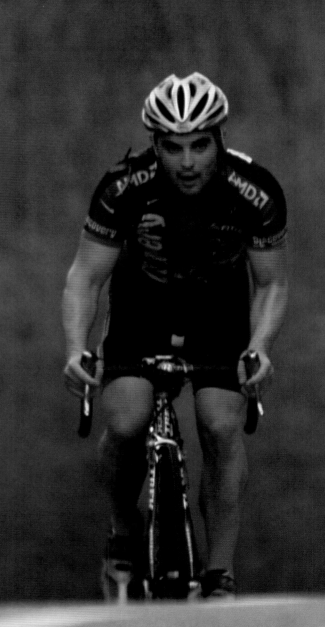

'The greatest tragedy
of the average man
is that he goes to his
grave with his music
still in him.'

Longfellow

Motivation

One of the best lecturers I've ever had was Steve Toadvine. His eternal phrase was one that I think we all should live by: 'Failing to plan is planning to fail.' Sit and think about the simplicity of this statement for a second and realise just how powerful it is. Whether you are aiming to climb Mount Everest, walk 4 miles, write your first book or get married, the same principles apply.

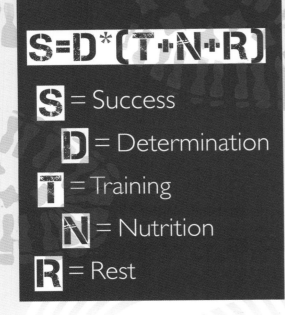

$$S = D * (T + N + R)$$

S = Success

D = Determination

T = Training

N = Nutrition

R = Rest

In this section, I am going to show you the way to achieve anything you want, not just in fitness, but in life – the approach is the same no matter what goal you want to achieve. People often ask me how I manage to finish the long-distance endurance events that I do each year, as they sound like huge achievements. I don't dispute that at all, they are great achievements, but they are simply long-term planning projects.

Take a marathon for instance – 26.2 miles. If I asked you to go out and run this distance tomorrow, chances are, you wouldn't be able to do it. But if I asked you to run it in 21 weeks and I broke down a training plan day by day, week by week, with a gradual increase each week to build up to doing a marathon, I am sure that I could get anyone across the line in a good time.

You see, most things seem unachievable at the start, but if you plan exactly how you are going to get there – weekly, monthly, yearly – then suddenly it becomes more attainable.

KARL'S TRUE LIFE STORY

Aged twenty-two, I sat in an exam hall in Smurfit Business School, stressed and unhealthy. I had taken out a €10,000 loan to pay for the course and as I sat there, shaking from stress, I put the paper down. I had a 'moment' where I looked at my life. I knew I had identified a gap in the market for a new business, I truly believed it could work. My gut instinct knew it could be done.

I reflected on the course I was doing and realised that it wasn't for me. Then, I did something that I had never ever done before, I pulled back my seat, stood up and walked out of the room containing several hundred people. I walked to the dean's office and told him that I wouldn't be coming back. With nerves and apprehension, yet with a sense of confidence, I walked out of the gates of Smurfit Business School realising the course wasn't for me, I had a plan in my mind and needed to get home to put it all down on paper, more than that, I had a good feeling about it, my gut instinct told me that this was the right way to go.

I went home, registered Karl Henry Personal Training, got out a large sheet of paper and began to brainstorm and plan, plan how I was going to get my business off the ground. My long-term goal was to have a bestselling fitness

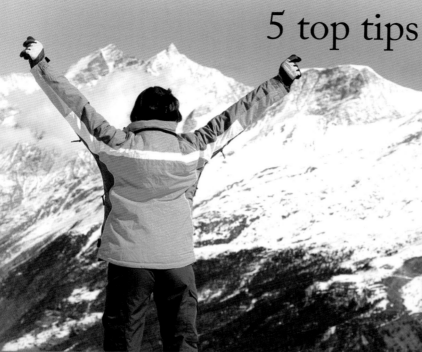

5 top tips for goal setting

▷ Believe in yourself when setting your goal.

▷ Write your goals down.

▷ Set new goals every 4 weeks.

▷ Place the goal somewhere visual, on your fridge or in your car.

▷ Every 4 weeks take a picture of something you have changed in the past 4 weeks that helped to work towards your goal.

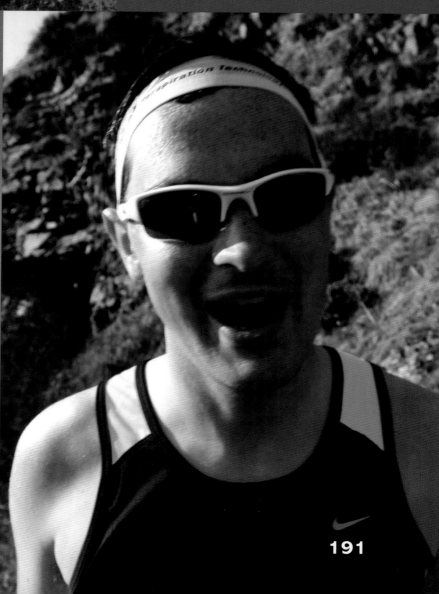

book. I gave myself five years to achieve this – and this is year six as I write. I broke my goals down into monthly targets for the number of clients I'd have, then media articles that I wanted to do and various other things. These all acted as building blocks towards further goals.

I haven't told you my story to massage my ego, but to show you that with the right planning anything can be achieved, don't let anyone tell you otherwise. No matter what your goal is, the 5 steps at the top of this page will help you achieve anything that you want to. So get that pen and paper out and let's get you to that goal. Are you ready? Here we go.

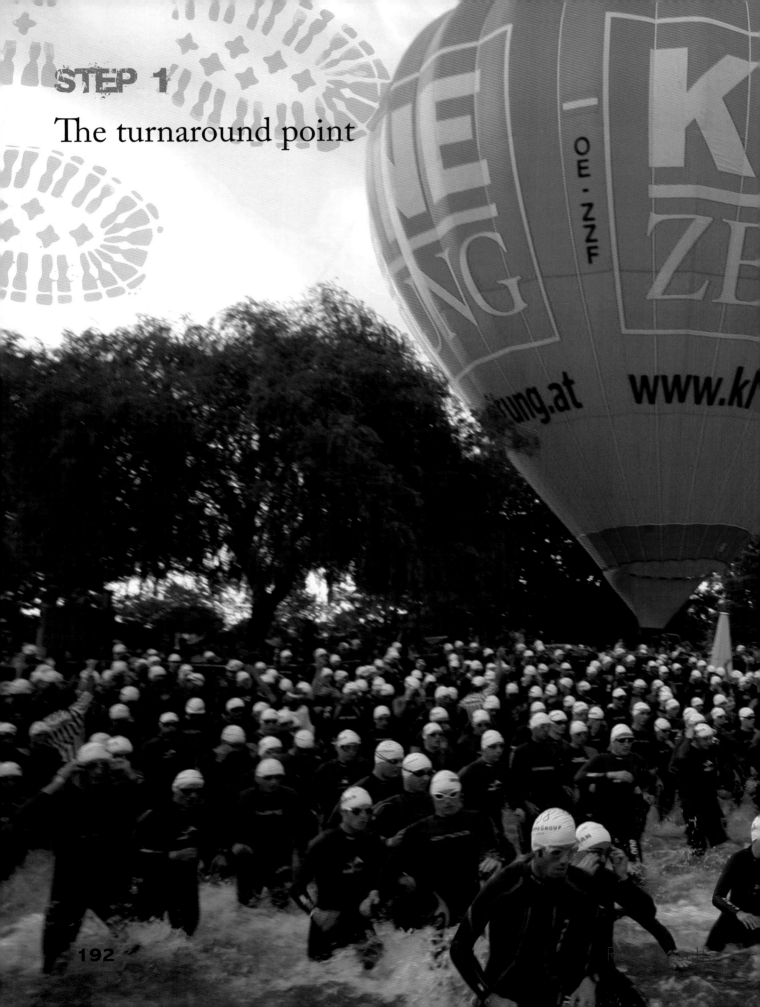

STEP 1

The turnaround point

This is the most important part of any goal-setting session. In my opinion, you need to hit this to get true focus. It might be looking at a photograph from your recent holiday, being unable to get into your favourite jeans or even sitting down at your desk realising that you no longer want to do the job that you are in, that you're bored and you want to change. You need to feel this sense of need, the need to change things in order to improve. By hitting this point, you will have the desire to make all the sacrifices needed and you won't be afraid to do make the change.

Before I train any new client, I always sit down with them for an informal chat, assessing their exercise and food background, etc. What I am really looking for is that need, hunger for assistance to help them lose that weight or run that marathon, whatever it may be. If you are trying to lose weight because your partner suggested it or for a similar reason, then it will make life an awful lot harder for you. You need to be doing this for you, not for anybody else. The desire has to come from you. With this desire, you will achieve the best results ever as you know why you are doing it. By reading this book, you will have all the information you will ever need to get into the best shape of your life – but all this information is futile unless you are doing it for you. When you have reached this point, you can move on to Step 2.

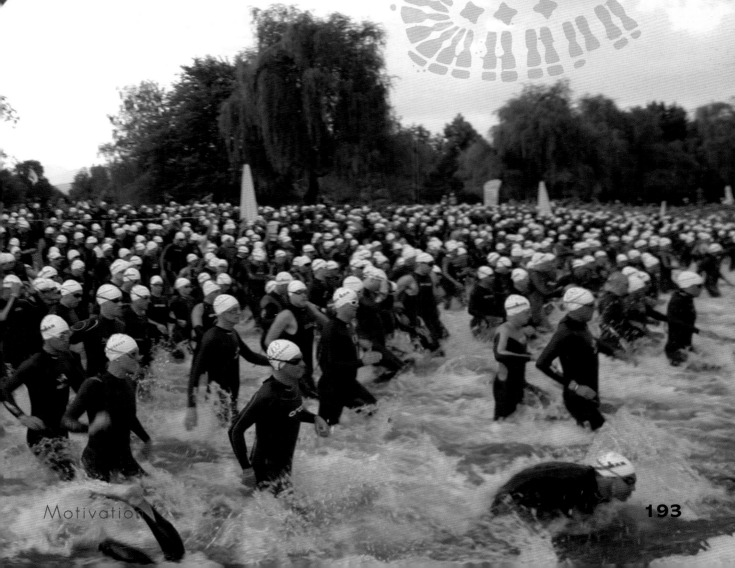

STEP 2 Setting the goal

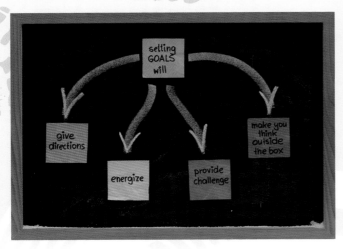

You have made the decision. Now comes the easy part, setting that goal. Many people are unsure just what the goal they are looking for is. To help with this, I always get people to take out a sheet of paper and write down the top five things they would like to achieve if they could achieve anything. No barriers to success whatsoever. This is important as it is easy to restrict yourself and you don't write down what it is you really want. Now that you have your top five goals on paper, I want you to list your top three. Think about it for a few minutes, of those five goals that you have in front of you, which are the most important to you? Well done! You are getting there. Now circle whichever goal jumps out at you, which one jumps off the page, screaming at you? This is the goal that you should pursue. This is the goal that you really want to achieve, that you are going to achieve. You must have that hunger in the pit of your stomach to achieve this goal, feel that desire as you look at it now.

STEP 3 Planning to reach the goal

Here is where I want you to make the contract. 'What contract?' I hear you say. The contract with yourself, that you are willing to do whatever it takes to achieve the goal you have set. This element of desire is important to get you to that point. On a personal level, I have missed numerous nights out, holidays and other things with my work schedule over the past few years, but these were sacrifices that I was willing to make and I don't regret any of them at all. I am not suggesting that you take things quite that far, but there will be some sacrifice that needs to be made, regardless of the goal. Maybe it's going out one night per week rather than two. Or changing that girls' meal out to a healthier restaurant rather than the one that you always go to. These are small changes that will make a big difference.

Before you start planning the goal, there is one other important factor in the equation – the people around you. Most of the time, I feel that the more people that you tell about your goal, the harder it is to achieve, and this is especially true in terms of weight loss. Unfortunately, this is also especially true for women. If you are a woman and trying to lose weight, then the fewer of your female friends you tell, the easier it will be for you to lose weight. I am not sexist in any way, shape or form, this is simply a something that I have found from experience.

On the other hand, if your goal is life changing in terms of work or in terms of time commitment to those around you, then you must sit down with those people and have them support you all the way. The fewer people that support you, the harder it will be for you to reach the goals that you have set for yourself. The more negative people that you have surrounding you, the harder it will be to achieve as they will, knowingly or unknowingly, pull the energy from you.

Now comes the actual planning. There are three ways in which you need to do this – short, medium and long term. Which one do you think is the most important? Which do you think that should be done first?

Always start with your long-term goals.

Long-term could be any length of time at all, 6 weeks to 6 years, it doesn't matter in terms of timescale. What matters is that this is your end goal, this is what you want to achieve. Now that you have your long-term goal in place, work back from it to your **medium-term** goal.

This should be the halfway point between today and achieving your goal. This acts to break down the mental frustration of having a goal that is too far away. If your goal is too far away, you may lose track of it and fall off the wagon. Your medium-term goals act to prevent this, by giving to something to focus on before the long-term goal. Now its time for the fun part, the short-term goals.

These act in exactly the same manner, breaking your goals down into a weekly and daily plans to achieve an overall goal. These are the bread and butter of any effective goal-setting plan.

Short-term plans make it easy to focus on your daily goals, eventually leading to the long-term goals over a period of time. Short-term goals are the foundations of the goal, a true essential component.

Type of goal	Time frame
Short term	Daily or weekly
Medium term	Halfway between the short term and long term
Long term	Any timescale – this should be your end result

Karl's Tips for Success

Fly with the eagles if you want to be an eagle yourself.

Don't surround yourself with negative people.

Don't be afraid to over plan this contract with yourself, the more detail you can put into it the better. Put it all down on paper and now walk away from it. Ideally, give yourself 24 hours away from the plan and then come back to it.

Is it still realistic?

Can it be done?

Is there anything that you would like to change?

If there is, well now is the time to do it, although obviously you can readjust your plan at any time. The most common mistake that is made at this point is that people aim to do too much. Remember that you need to have balance in the plan, by aiming to do too much, you may just tire yourself out!

STEP 4 Tips to keep you going

I feel that this is often the most important part of overall goal setting. By having your short-term goals, you are giving yourself constant ways to monitor your progress. When you achieve these goals, you should treat yourself, reward yourself. Say, for example, your goal is to go the gym three times a week for the first four weeks and you achieve this. Well, grab that handbag or your wallet and off you go – treat yourself. Now it doesn't have to be something big, it's just the process so that you feel good about achieving your goal, and so you should feel good about it!

Another great tip is that if you get thrown off course, just get straight back on the wagon. Life is a rollercoaster as we know, sometimes things come up that you won't have planned for. Simply accept that these things have happened and get back on track, don't dwell on them, just put them behind you and move on to next week's goals.

Make sure that you have left enough time for yourself to rest and recover from your sessions. Often people aim to do too much in their plans and they burn themselves out, the way to get around this is simply to rest up as required in your plan.

Why not print off a photo of your goal and make it visual? I do this with brides who come into me to get in shape for their weddings. I get to see a photo of the dress and get them to keep one at their computer, in their handbag or even in their car. By making your goal visual, you can see what you are working towards, making it a whole lot easier for you. I won't even begin to tell you some of the goal photos that I have seen over the years, but let's just say that you can make any goal visual.

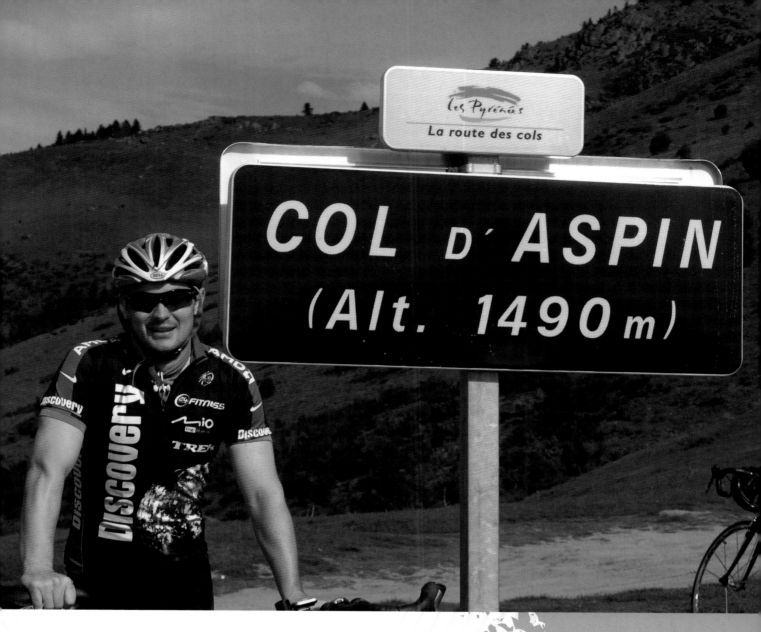

If you find that you aren't reaching your goal, don't worry, it is not time to pack it all in. I never see failure as a negative thing, you just need to go back to your plan and change it so that it will work for you, using all your experience from the first time round. How are you meant to get experience if you don't try something? Never view failure as a negative thing, ever. I have failed to complete two ironman triathlons, collapsing twice. Yet I have no regrets whatsoever about either of the races, I learned so much from both and will use that experience in preparing better for the next one that I am doing. If you don't try to achieve something, you will never know if you could have done it or not!

Karl's Tips for Success

Take charge of your life.

Create your future.

Clarify your values.

Determine your true goals.

STEP 5 A new goal

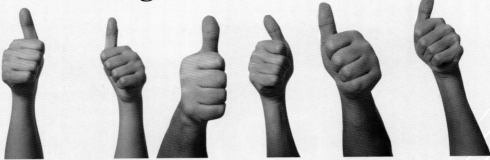

Yes! You are there, that long-term goal has become a reality. What seemed so far away has come more quickly than you expected. You are there. Slimmer, fitter, in a new job, whatever it was, you are now there. Don't forget to treat yourself, we know how important that is.

When you have done that, the next step is to start the whole process all over again. Your goals this time may be totally different, but you are giving your body and your mind something to work towards. The ability to be working towards something is key to achieving long-term success when it comes to your goals. It is when you become static that you might find yourself going backwards, which is never good. But by sticking to the very same formula, the same method, you will ensure that you are working towards your true goals, those goals that you really want to get.

	Goal	Time frame	How
Long-term goal	Lose 1 stone	6 weeks	3 gym sessions p/w
Medium-term goal	Lose 7 pounds	3 weeks	3 gym sessions p/w
Short-term goal	Lose 2 pounds	1 week	3 gym sessions p/w

Failure is a positive

We have all been there, a race or a goal or something in life that just hasn't worked out as planned. You had the courage to try something and it didn't work. All too often people can beat themselves up over situations like this, feeling that they have failed, that they are a failure and then they proceed to get down about it.

Guess what? Failure is a good experience, because you had the guts, the bravery to try something, to strive to achieve something that so many others didn't.

No matter at what stage you didn't achieve you still learned so much about yourself and the goal that you had in mind. If you hadn't tried, then you would be left pondering the 'what-if' scenario – and it's far worse to feel like that, than to have failed at something. You can then use all that you have learned to plan a different approach to achieving that goal. Why not go for it again? A great man once said, 'If you fail at first, then try, try again', and this is so true.

Real Results

The five P's of effective planning

Simple yet effective, these tips will ensure that your plan is the best that it can be, helping you to work towards your goals better.

Purpose What is your goal? What are you working towards?

Passion In order to achieve your goal, you must be passionate about it and be ready to work hard towards it.

Planning Just as I showed you above, plan step by step about how you are going to get to your goal.

Perspiration There will be sweat, blood and tears I am sure, but these will be required to get you to your goal.

Perserverance As always, situations will get in your way but you must persevere and work around these obstacles that get in your way. This is one of the most important parts as so often people fall off the bandwagon when something negative or unexpected happens.

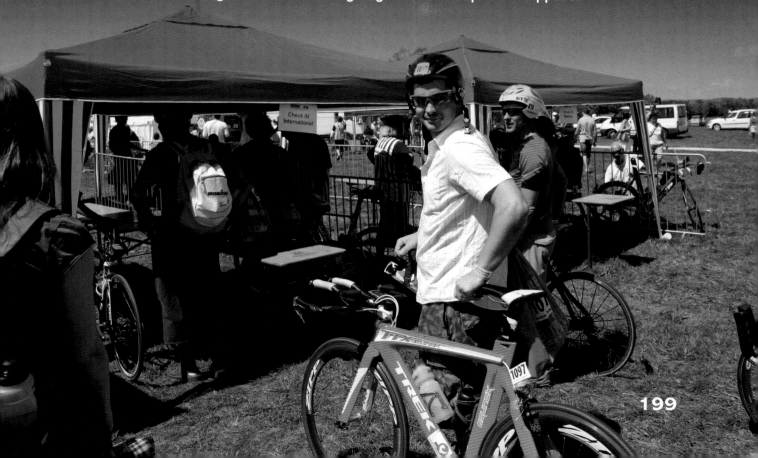

It took me many marathons to get under the 4-hour mark, a lot of times I thought that I had done enough and that I would break the time that I had set for myself, each and every time that I didn't hit my goal I learned something new, some new training tip and some new method. These things that I have learned have been invaluable in my career, without having continued to try break that time, I never would have learned them.

I am a firm believer that you must learn by doing, no matter what courses claim to do, they just don't give you the same as experience in life. Every year, I set myself new goals and new sports to continue my education in life, if I don't achieve the goals that I set out to do, I continue to train and change until I achieve them. Don't sit on your backside beating yourself up, look at all you have learned, all the positive elements that have been created by your aiming to achieve, now try to plan out a different method of getting there, using all your knowledge and go for it again. Keep going, we all hit road blocks on the way, but you will never know unless you try.

I want to use a quotation by Theodore Roosevelt, who was the twenty-sixth US president, to sum my feelings on failure up.

> *"It is not the critic who counts; not the man who points out how the strong man stumbles, or where the doer of deeds could have done them better. The credit belongs to the man who is actually in the arena, whose face is marred by dust and sweat and blood, who strives valiantly; who errs and comes short again and again; because there is not effort without error and shortcomings; but who does actually strive to do the deed; who knows the great enthusiasm, the great devotion, who spends himself in a worthy cause, who at the best knows in the end the triumph of high achievement and who at the worst, if he fails, at least he fails while daring greatly. So that his place shall never be with those cold and timid souls who know neither victory nor defeat."*

> Theodore Roosevelt *(1858–1919), from*
> *'Man in the Arena' speech given 23 April 1910*

If ever you needed a push to go for something again, just read Roosevelt's words again, sit for a while and listen to the words, feel the passion in his writing and be stirred by what you read, be motivated to get back on track again.

I am an avid reader of success and motivational books. I have been lucky enough to see many of the world's best speakers and to learn from them. While I am totally against the cult formation that surrounds some of these speakers, there are some great tips to be taken from what they have to say. Below is a sample of some of the tips that I have used and that I think have a universal appeal for everyone. No flowery language, just straight-to-the-point ideas that will help you on your journey.

Real Results

Mind mapping

There are so many ways to find your goals, these can often become confusing. One of the easiest and most effective ways of finding out exactly what your goal is, is called mind mapping. Often used to study or memorise big blocks of information, mind mapping is so easy to do and I have found it extremely effective with many of my clients.

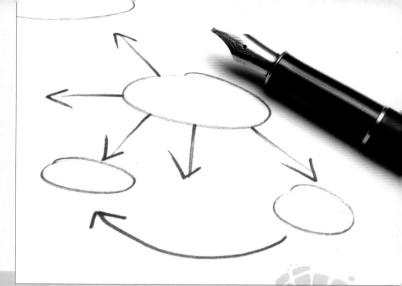

Follow these simple steps and see how you get on.

▷ Sit down at your table with a blank sheet of paper in front of you.

▷ In the centre of the page, write ME and draw a circle around it.

▷ From this, draw strands to any words that come into your mind, I want you to write down everything that comes into your head, and just keep drawing the strands.

▷ This is also called a brain dump, literally get all the information out of your mind and on paper.

▷ Now, here is the important part, walk away from the page and leave it until the next morning.

▷ Take a different coloured pen and circle the key words that jump out at you.

▷ Slowly but surely, you will see exactly what is important to you in terms of your goals, your true goals.

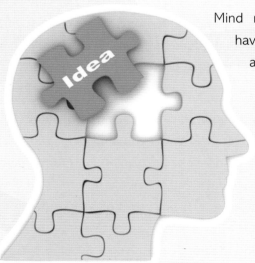

Mind mapping works, no question about it. I have used it personally both when studying and when planning my own goals. It only works though if you are totally honest with yourself when writing everything down, leave no stone unturned and empty out all of your thoughts. The more you write down the more benefit you will get from it, I promise. I know just how scary it can be!

Visualisation

An important tool in business and sport, visualisation is just a powerful tool to help you lose weight and achieve your goals. I am aware that it sounds scary to some people, and can seem intimidating or just down right stupid, but neglect it at your peril. The good news is that it does not involve any meditation or yoga-based breathing in case that scares you!

Visualisation is simply seeing yourself as you want to be. No matter what your goal is, you need to visualise it. I often tell my clients to do this just before they go to sleep, as it is possibly the best time to do it. As you close your eyes to go to sleep, just imagine your goal in your mind. Let's say for example it's your first marathon race. Imagine yourself at the start line, how does it feel? How are you feeling? Try to feel the sensations that you are going to feel on the day, your muscles, your position in the starting line up. Now listen to the gun going off, your beginning to run, how are your legs? At the halfway point now, imagine yourself being positive, feeling good, enjoying the race and continue this all the way through until you get to the end, feel yourself crossing the finish line and all the emotions that you will feel. This is basically creating a blueprint for your race.

I have met athletes who use this technique when they are injured and actually come back better than they were before the injury, that is how powerful it is.

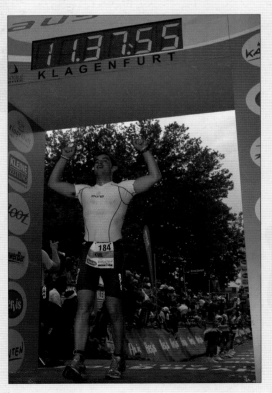

If you feel that this is too much for you, there are other and easier ways to do it. Simply pull out a picture of how you want to look, be it one of you in your past or someone in a magazine that you strive to look like. Put these pictures in places that you can see them, your diary, desk or even your fridge. You want to see these every day, as this is what you are working towards, this is what you want to be. Rather than not being able to describe it, you now have a picture of it, just try it to see how this changes your results!

All in all, motivation is one of the keys to success. Without having a goal, it is very hard to see where you are going. Without that clarity, it is so much harder to keep training long term. Many of the methods that I have outlined here will be new to you, but what have you got to lose by not trying them? As with anything that I recommend, they are simple techniques that work – otherwise I wouldn't have included them. So go on, get out that paper, put down those goals, start working towards them and keep using the tips to keep yourself on track!

Appendix

In this section, I want to give you all the best websites and books that you can use to help you on the road to being eating more healthily and getting more exercise.

Websites

www.mapmyrun.com A great website that helps you check the distance of your runs and get all the information you would ever need from your sessions — best of all its free!

www.garmin.com Garmin provide some of the best equipment for sports, tracking speed, distance and heart-rate monitors.

www.amphibianking.com Damien in Amphibian King was the first to offer gait analysis, there are now several shops offering this service.

www.irishfit.eu Irish Fit is fantastic for clothing and training gear.

www.lifestylesports.com Lifestyle Sports is a 100 per cent Irish-owned company, operating 65 sports outlets spread across Ireland and Northern Ireland and offers quality clothing and gait analysis in many of its stores. Many thanks to Lifestyle for providing the clothing for many of the photos in this book.

www.runireland.com This is one of the best websites around for getting to know the racing calendar in Ireland. There is also fantastic advice on offer from many people involved in the running scene.

www.wheelworxbikes.com Rob Cummins has created Ireland's utopia of triathlon stores. This is the biggest triathlon store in the country, with so much experience Rob can give you so much advice too.

www.activeeurope.com This website has all the races all over Europe. No matter what it is you want to do, you can find a race to try.

www.magicseaweed.com All the surfing information all across the country — and across the world. Simply put in your location and view all the latest information, including the best time to get the waves.

www.trekbikes.com All my bikes are by TREK and I can't recommend them enough. If they are good enough for Lance Armstrong, they are good enough for me!

www.ironguides.com I have used Ironguides as my coach for Ironman and ultra-marathon races, they are the best there is, up to date and providing the best training plans there are.

www.triathlonireland.com The website for the Irish Triathlon Federation — everything there is to know about the Irish triathlon scene.

www.surfcoachireland.ie Richie Fitzgerald is the best surf coach in the country, with a great store in Bundoran, County Sligo. He will have you standing up on the board in no time — or if you are looking to improve your surfing, he will have you surfing 20 foot waves in no time!

www.isasurf.ie If surfing is something you have just started, this website will teach you the rules of the beach as well as all the safety tips.

www.coillte.ie Coillte have done amazing work in the past couple of years all around the country for walking trails, mountain biking and hiking trails. Their website has maps of all their trails around the country and everything you need to know.

www.lululemon.com This is some of the most comfortable, trendy and cool training and yoga gear on the planet, it can be expensive but it's worth it.

www.terroirs.ie Sean and Francoise run this fabulous business and will get you sorted with the best organic wines.

www.underarmour.com Under Armour is the best brand for tough training gear, running clothing and chilled-out training gear. I have been using their clothing for a long time and it's the best I have found. Especially their winter training clothes, seriously warm!

www.paulamee.com I have worked with Paula over the years and have no doubt that she is the best nutritionist in the country. No matter what question you have, Paula will put you on the right track.

www.jellyfishsurfco.com A great surf shop in Clonakilty, I bought my first board here and shop here when I am in West Cork.

www.macnallyopticians.com If you want to train hard, you need some good sunglasses to protect your eyes. Ellen and Kevin have looked after my clients and myself over the years from their premises on St Stephen's Green.

www.medicosmeticcentre.com I always recommend my clients to Catherine if they are looking to get a colonic done. I think Catherine is the best in the country and I have seen clients getting great results with her.

www.travelpaths.com I always use Anna to organise my flights and travel arrangements to races and other events. In this digital age, many people don't use travel agents but from my experience this group is fantastic!

Books

I am passionate about reading and read as often as I can. Below are just some of the books that I think readers of this book just might enjoy.

Born to Run, Christopher McDougall

Brother Iron/Sister Steel, Dave Draper

Building the Classic Physique, Steve Reeves

Chew on This, Eric Schlosser

Cinderella Man, Melinda Delisa

Fat Land, Greg Critzer

Fat Wars, Ellen Ruppell Shell

Going Long, Joe Friel and Gordo Byrne

It's not About the Bike, Lance Armstrong

Le Tour, Geoffrey Wheatcroft

Look Your Best, Tara King

Not on the Label, Felicity Lawrence

No Limits, Michael Phelps

Rough Ride, Paul Kimmage

Running Commentary, Frank Grealy

South, Col Wilfred Noyce

South, Ernest Shackleton

The Art of Happiness, Dalai Lama

The Omnivores' Dilemma, Michael Pollan

What I Talk About When I Talk About Running, Murakimi